WHERE TO START

LIVING AND COPING
WITH A DISABILITY

ALEXANDAR CAMPION

An ***abled <u>wheelchair</u> user

Copyright © Alexandar Campion 2023.

The right of Alexandar Campion to be identified as the author of this work has been asserted in accordance with the Copyright, Designs and Patents Act 1988.

All rights reserved. No part of this publication may be reproduced, stored in or transmitted into any retrieval system, in any form, or by any means (electronic, mechanical, photocopying, recording or otherwise) without the prior written permission of the publisher. Any person who does any unauthorised act in relation to this publication may be liable to criminal prosecution and civil claims for damages.

The images in this book are almost entirely the author's collection.

Every attempt has been made to gain permission for the use of images not from the author's collection in this book.

Any omissions will be rectified in future editions.

ISBN: 978-1-913012-90-8

Published in partnership with Chalk Stream Books
(an imprint of Riverside Publishing Solutions).

Printed and bound in the UK.

CONTENTS

Introduction		v
About The Author		ix
1.	Dealing with the trauma	1
2.	Your needs now from your body and listening to them	9
3.	Care basics & pressure sores	14
4.	Eating and drinking	19
5.	Help	25
6.	The somewhat stupid questions you get asked	33
7.	Adaptions for the home and daily life	39
8.	OTs, physios, doctors and psychologists	46
9.	Impact on family and friends	52
10.	Making your schedule	61
11.	Learning your energy levels	65
12.	The perks of the chair	71
13.	The paperwork	74
14.	Finances	76
15.	Clothing	79
16.	Changes to look out for	81
17.	Finding your new interests and hobbies or working out a way to carry on with old ones	85
18.	Brain food	91
19.	Sex. Yes!	94

20.	Sharing	98
21.	Social and work situations	102
22.	Movement and exercise	104
23.	Travelling	108
24.	Things that just make life a little easier	112
25.	Psychology of your own making	113
26.	Breakthrough treatments, news and Google	116
27.	Helpful links	118
28.	The diagrams of movement	121
29.	Summary	133
30.	Back of the book: What you can do?	134

INTRODUCTION

Where to start? Well, I think a fair warning about this book and its content. If you want a book that is going to cuddle you and tell you everything will be OK and not have some short, hard-hitting stuff, e.g. straight down the line; no BS approach, then pop it back on the shelf.

If however you really want to know the truth behind the chair and its implications on you or your family member/s or friends then read on. However, I want to be as clear as humanly possible. If you read this and then think you will know everything about disability – you won't. Bear in mind, this is only from my perspective. For a start, everyone is different, and every disability varies and has its own challenges.

What I am offering you if you're the person in the position of being in a wheelchair for life or have suffered a spinal cord injury like me is simple. Well to a degree, as life isn't going to be as simple as it was! Within this book you will find:

- A no BS approach to spinal cord injury and disability.
- Wheelchair life; the tricks that keep you out of hospital.
- Tips to not get caught out and how to be prepared.
- The way I live my life and my perspective, which I keep getting told is certainly very different.

With this, understand I can only speak of my own experiences and give you what I have learnt and what I have also learnt from others. This I feel has to be without the layer of worrying about hurting your feelings. It will be straight down the line, and I will be blunt but if you're still reading maybe it's just what you need. I wish I had had a book like this when I was first adapting to life with a disability as I like to deal with the situation (i.e. the problems) and find in my opinion, the best solutions.

Lastly, to people not in wheelchairs: don't think this book will help you understand everything fully. It provides insight, a different perspective, methodology, and the details given are definitely not the 'standard' approach or the standard for disability in general.

Re-reading this I found there was a massive point I need to make off the bat. If you are dealing with disability or spinal cord injury like mine and in a wheelchair, have a lower limb disability for life or even a short while, here are some key points:

- To become as independent as possible.
- Study your medication/s; know the shape and size of the pills you are taking.
- Make sure you know how things work on your chair or walking aids and have an understanding of these things.

Basically, you need a strong base of knowledge really quickly to become independent as smoothly and safely as possible. I hope to be able to provide insight into this.

In the spinal unit I went to which will remain unnamed, I was given someone else's meds twice (which would have killed me) and was nearly given ten times the dosage of another medication that would have had me shitting for days! I was also sadly assaulted verbally and physically by a nurse crossing a line.

Yeah, they didn't get away with it and were subsequently fired. There's a line. You and only you can be responsible for that line and for yourself. Even if you are stuck in a bed, you can control things – meds, food, the way you are treated and your independence. That is your lifeline. And that is why I wrote this book.

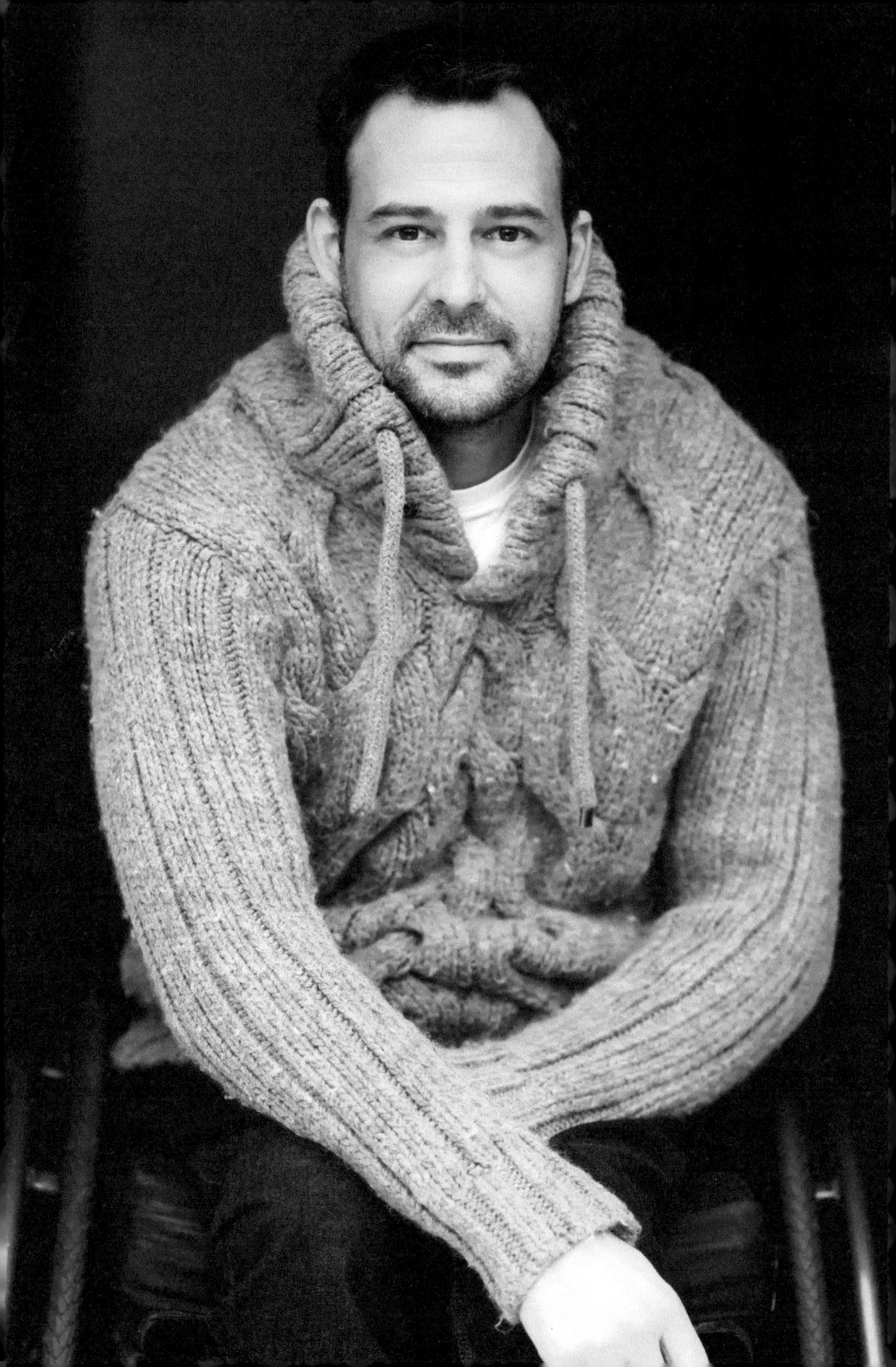

ABOUT THE AUTHOR

Me. My name is Alexandar Campion. I sound like I'm starting a bloody Alcoholics Anonymous meeting but I'm not; I'm telling you who I am and why on this God's green earth I have any reason to offer advice. Well, I'm coming up to my tenth year on wheels. (Actually, I am finishing this in late 2022, so it has now been a decade)

I am a category A T-6 paraplegic, which in-short means I can feel everything above the bottom of my ribcage/nipple area upwards.

I can't use or feel my legs, but I can feel them with my hands(!) and I use them to get up off the floor — don't worry, I will explain that later.

So I ended up in a wheelchair from an 8mph tip off a motorbike. Yes, not 80 or 180... 8mph. (Grrrr)

You know, I was more pissed off with that than actually breaking my back, but that's the way it goes. Ironically and funnily enough, it's actually called a chance fracture.

I was wearing full gear, e.g. helmet, leathers, boots and a spine protector. Where my back actually broke was T12-L1, but the lucky man I am, I hit rubber and also broke 13 ribs, crushed T6,7,8,9 vertebrae, sliced my liver and got a good bump on the head giving me a subdural haematoma (brain bleed). I was told by the surgeon putting me back together that if I had only hit the curb, I only would have broken a collar bone. I believe I said, "Good to know that for next time."

Subsequently, *this is why I cringe at cyclists and motorcyclists not wearing the right gear... 8mph!*

Yes, I had every intention on getting back on a bike and getting back to university, and I did but that's a story for later.

Why have I written this? Well, I have found that people are either too scared to say what I am going to, or won't as they live in a bubble of what they have been told that they can and cannot do.

Now this, from a medical perspective is kind of true and sort of a way of locking you into a way of thinking and also a set lifestyle, which it doesn't need to be.

In no way am I saying all guidelines are wrong, I just think some of it is outdated and now not very relevant. It's a hell of a lot of red tape, ass-covering within that system. Also the fact that once you're in your lovely wheelchair (yes, a tone of sarcasm) there are ways to stop yourself getting ripped off left right and centre, and YES living life again with a strong dash of being independent and free.

About me; I'm 36, I work in design and engineering, and I've been exceptionally lucky with my life and found out the short cuts to use with my wheelchair – sometimes the hard way! But also, by asking older wheelchair users the best or easiest ways to live in a wheelchair.

I don't view myself as disabled or "handy-capable" (whoever made up that dumb-ass term isn't 'handy-capable'!)

I get on with it and find ways of doing things. I am just me; my perspective has changed not just because of my height since being in a wheelchair (lol!). Well maybe on a couple of small things, but I am pleased to say I'm still the same stubborn, slightly crazy git I was before my accident, and I'm OK with that.

Please note: I am not a medical professional and on any of the below, I would consult your doctor or consultant.

1. DEALING WITH THE TRAUMA

OH FUCK!

Yeah, these were the first words that came out of my mouth when I was first injured. Obscene I know, but given the situation, I hope you understand.

I felt down my leg and knew I had fucked myself up as I couldn't feel my legs or move them. I knew there and then.

A few moments after waking, my dad was by my bedside. We waited for the surgeon to come in and tell me just how badly screwed I was. Turns out pretty bad.

I had done a proper job; so I was right: I had broken my back.

As you know or guess the first question I asked was,

"Will I walk again; 0–100?" Reply, "Zero." OK. The second I asked was, "Where did you study?" He told me. I said, "OK. Can you hold out your hands?" "OK thanks, I wanted to see if they were steady." He was going to be poking around in my spine after all.

At this point I won't lie, I bawled my eyes out the moment he had left the room, and my dad did too for the next 20 minutes. Then as we started to stop I said, "Hey, it's not all bad – free parking now!"

We both burst out laughing and a mixture of irony and stupid jokes followed from this point on, and they've never stopped.

The saying, *'sometimes you have to laugh or cry'* has never been more true.

I knew what I had done. I also know this one key point: If you are riding a bike or doing some stupid shit that will lead you to get hurt, don't go bloody moaning about it. Take it on the chin and deal with it. Some find this view hard to accept but it is nonetheless true in my opinion. Self-blame and regret isn't helpful but accepting it and owning it – well, that changes the whole picture. Note: acceptance.

Trauma in all people is different. However, the above was my experience. Now I believe the best thing was understanding the injury itself.

Days after my operation to put me back together and as soon as the pain medication (morphine) had cleared out of my system, my mind was clearer, and I would study what had happened. I asked a lot of questions, not only about my injury but the full picture – how, why, what, what it means?

I was always told to slow down and that I would learn in time (probably because I was in a general hospital). I didn't accept that.

I had by this point accepted it and gathered enough information to understand that I would more than likely be in the chair for life. I immediately thought, "OK, how am I going to get back on my bike and back to uni?"

I had to tell the hospital priest and counsellor to politely f**k off plenty of times, as apparently 'I wasn't dealing with the loss of use of my legs in the **right way**'. Both of these people seemed to be in perfect health and walking... lol.

Sorry to both of them, but they really were just that annoying. I don't need to be told how I was supposed to be feeling.

The priest took it well and she sent me a post card a few days later saying, "I would agree with you if you were right" written on the front. On the back was a nice message just saying, "I saw this and thought of you. Keep it up," with a smiley face.

Now, understanding your injury and its ramifications for you are really important but this does take 2–3 years to set in. By that, I mean your body adjusts to your injury and your mental state as your brain re-wires.

Some parts will heal, and some will not. Keeping hope that you might heal is good, but realistically if you are complete, (like me, a category A paraplegic) it is very rare. Small changes happen and it's important to look out for them and if found, work them as much as possible.

Note: Understanding spinal cord injury is such a specific field of study and even though you may be able to understand the broad strokes of the medical terminology and the implications, I believe *you will learn more though listening to your own body.*

Warning – false hope: Clinical studies with stem cells and gels that can slow the spinal cord from healing are all years in development and still not in clinical human trails. I must have had ten texts the day they got a sausage dog to walk again! This was a step forward for the science, but I know it won't be for me (both figuratively and literally!)

What I could do was accept it and roughly understand how it was going to be for me, and that's exactly what I did. I was able to adapt I would say quicker, to my new life in a wheelchair. I think it was about a week after my operation, I was shown how to transfer safely into a chair. I got told off within an hour for trying to back wheel balance in my chair, but hey I wanted to do wheelies!

Acceptance is an odd thing and I have been told by many people from doctors to nurses to OTs (occupational therapists) and psychologists that I should expect a downer!? Moment or depression in my mood. But I think accepting it with limited understanding, helped me live my life without yet having the 'downer moment'. I still never give up hope of change or improvement but also live with my current reality of being in a wheelchair.

Carl Rogers is a psychologist who writes about acceptance and understanding and the paradox this can present. For the most part however, I deal with life in the moment and plan for the future.

I will tell people what happened and guess at the questions I or you will undoubtedly be asked over and over and preparing my answers to speed along the conversation as to be honest, I can't travel back in time and deal with a 'what if I just' or 'if I had just'. There is no time machine or magic fix or currently no treatment out there that will get you out the chair, but never give up on the hope. Personally I do hope medical treatment radically shifts, but I don't bank on it happening within my lifetime. I do stay as fit as possible and keep myself in check with dealing with my own physical and emotional thoughts towards how I am feeling – this would be the hope.

In essence the physiology for everybody is different and my way may not be yours; some choose to take the time to grieve and some wallow in it. I personally didn't and don't see the point, as try as you might – you can't change it, no matter what Google articles have come up saying stem cell treatment is going to be available shortly. I read these same articles at the time of my injury. They still exist today and I'm writing this a decade later. *Hard fact is, just dust off, pick up and move forward.* Hard to hear but it is that simple. This is my own approach and personal view on it.

Points: This is vital to get your head around – the time it takes to hurt yourself or be injured is in my view, half the time you should take to adapt and accept it.

You can take the time to wallow later or even have regrets but at the moment you are told – no, it's game on.

You have to pick up, crack on and push through, learn quickly and adapt yourself even quicker. This is the biggest challenge and is explained how to do this in later chapters.

If you do not adapt to the change as quickly as you can and respond to the trauma of the base injury you can fall even further both physically and mentally. I think this will be argued but hey, this is just my personal opinion, and everyone is different. By no means am I shaming other ways or approaches.

First – Accept you will hate it, resent it but hell if you can't change it, accept it, and make gains, there is very little you can do to change it all. You may be in a position to get improvement but let's say you're busy thinking, looking back and wallowing, you miss out on that vital window and fall further down. This is what I would avoid at all costs.

Second – Learn, learn, learn – listen to your doctors and consultants. The advice you are given by the people around you, e.g. medical professionals – learn it, document it, and act upon it. Take the time to get the basic understanding of medical terminology. A pen and paper come in handy or a recorder so you can re-listen to conversations which can really help later in adapting all or parts of the information given and then apply what you feel is relevant and correct for you – the individual.

Third – Don't be afraid to ask the stupid questions about your injury or illness and also don't be afraid to question the opinions of those offering advice. After all everything is subjective, even my view here.

Fourth – The environment you are in. Make it your space as much as possible to have something that grounds you. Whether that's a photo of a place you want to visit, a goal written down or a memory, don't give in because of your situation. Everything is certainly not over; it is simply just finding new ways to achieve as much independence as possible. This helped me and I started small. Find one thing then work on the next and so on. Just keep setting new goals, tasks, and you do adapt and for lack of a better term, problem solve and therefore move forward with your new path that you are building for yourself.

Lastly – Social media, friends and family. Contact with people may be tricky. It is important to control this flow and set your own rules of who you want around and what you want to be looking at. For me, I cut off interactions while rehabilitating in my new life. In part this was maybe to get my head straight. In other ways, I didn't want the distraction or the fuss/attention. I put up a few posts on social media to let people know I was OK, but I wasn't wanting to see anyone. I think for me this was a good idea as it allowed me to move quicker through the system and not have to explain to others the full details; bearing in mind I was still trying to understand them myself. So family and friends were out. I had very few visits and when I did, it was towards the end of my stay or I kept visits short so I could limit the conversation flow, etc.

Now, these five points are a personal perspectives and were key for me and me alone. I wanted to get in and out of hospital/spinal centre as quickly as possible, bear that in mind. Also, this isn't a one-size-fits-all guide, but it is only a perspective – physically and psychologically. Was it right or wrong? Well, I'm still kicking and not moaning and haven't been back in hospital so, I would say it was a win. Was it healthy? In the next ten years, maybe I will find out.

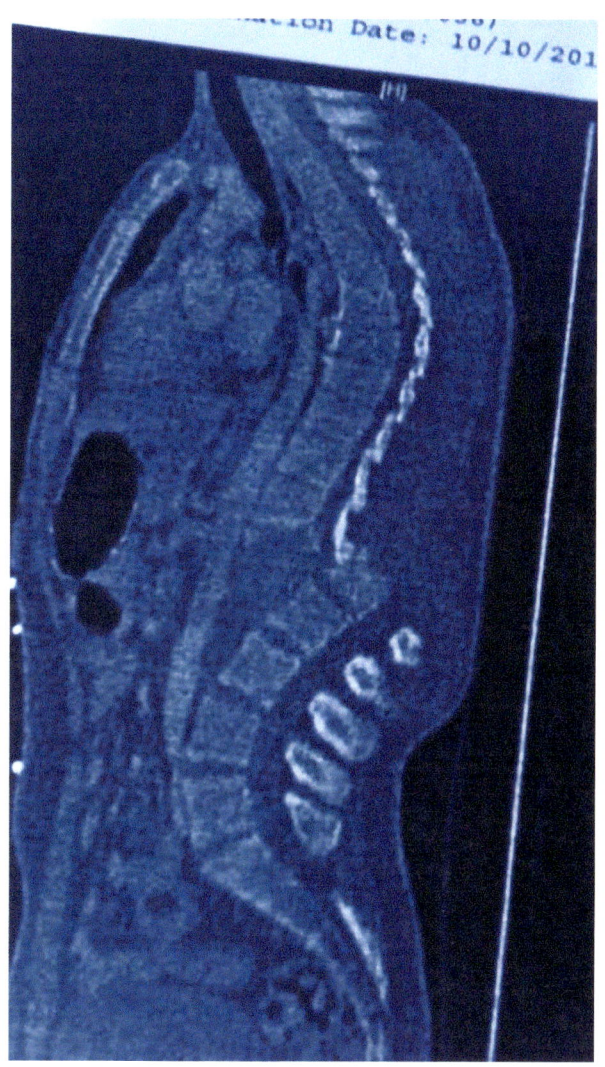

YEAH, THIS IS REALLY BROKEN!

Here above you see the X-ray of my spine. So your vertebrae are supposed to look like nice square blocks. As you can see, top moving down T6,7,8,9,10 are like bricks and then T12-L1 is where the spinal cord was severed. The spinal cord sits in the gap between the blocks and the white dots to the right of them. (See diagram on next page).

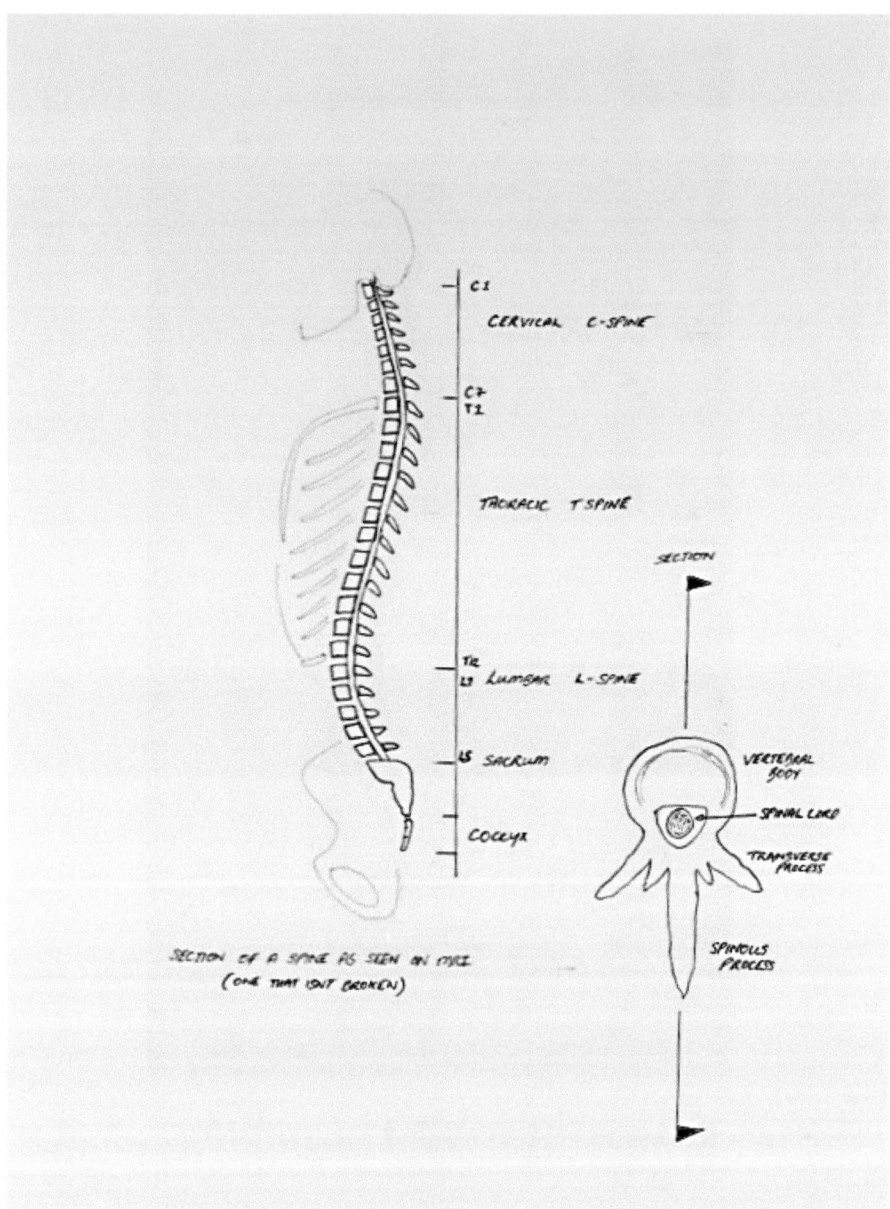

What it should look like! E.g. ... not broken.

2. YOUR NEEDS FROM YOUR BODY NOW AND LISTENING TO THEM

Spasms: For myself, I get stomach spasms which I have learnt can mean a few things:

1. I need to pee or use the loo. Yep, my stomach will start to move of its own accord.
2. **Pain or injury:** You can't feel it but this can still trigger them.
3. **Stress:** It's your brain sending signals to your legs to walk away but the wire has been cut, so the signal ends up there. (I'm referring to my spinal cord.)

Note: The best way I have had the spinal cord explained to me is it's the thickness of a little finger that goes from the brain to the coccyx and slightly beyond it like rubber bands twisted together. If you nip it, it will fray and you can't just tie them back together, Also it is 120 billion (yes, billion!) rubber bands all carrying electrical input/output signals from your brain to your limbs. Now those signals have to end somewhere, so all being well it would send the message to your foot. Then your foot would lift but when you have either severed or damaged it, the signals end at this point causing a spasm.

4. **Hydration/Dehydration:** Drinking or lack of drinking something or very warm and very cold drinks can cause the same type of spasm. This is easier to identify and the same also can happen with a change in air temperature and also food.

If you're wondering what spasms feels like, get a slender tone belt, attach it to your tummy, turn it onto full and hit on and off in rapid succession. Not pleasant but can be a useful way of explaining it to others. Also, the belt can be used to reduce spasms, but I will touch on this later in chapter 17.

What do spasms do? Well, mine cause me to lurch over to the left or right. I get them on the left side of my abdominal muscles and right of my back. This is because where my spine was damaged, it's not a straight cut-off point or a clear line of loss of sensation. This is useful as I can trigger muscles that are able to work for me and exercise them to help with balance. Also, when a spasm hits, I cope with it by breathing deeply (or trying to!) and then checking which of the four above could be the cause.

Headaches: As you're not designed or made to sit down all day, headaches are commonplace. Therefore, on a fundamental level, standing using a standing frame can help, but you generally feel like utter shit when you do. This is because your heart is working harder, and your blood pressure drops and whatever you do to kill the boredom is a necessary evil.

I personally hate it, so I don't do as much as I should (naughty boy, as I'm told, lol), but it helps with blood pressure, heart health and slows down osteoporosis (which is where bones become weaker from not load-bearing because of all the sitting). Other reasons for headaches can be pain in an area you can't feel, injury, dehydration, non-movement and not moving around enough.

Warning about headaches: They can be a precursor sign of something much more serious which is called Autonomic dysreflexia – (AD) a disorder of the spinal reflex activity occurring in those with a spinal cord injury such as mine. It can be a sudden onset hypertension, sweating, bradycardia and headache. If left unchecked, this can lead to death in simple terms. In very simple terms, it is where the spinal cord is damaged is not allowing it to process nerve signals correctly. It can mean many things but if you have a headache that is splitting and you're sweating and cannot find a problem, seek medical attention without thinking. You may be over-reacting better but better to be safe than sorry, and never wait too long.

Twitches: Now these are not like spams and I could deliberately find areas to voluntarily move and other areas that would do it on their own. It can be a slightly odd feeling to see something move but not have full sensation of it.

Neuropathic pain: This is a complex field for me as I have hypersensitivity around my torso. Again this is different for everyone, but mine feels like a tight band around my chest 2–3 inches in width, which consistently feels like sunburn. (This is the best way I have found to explain it to others.)

I can block it out mentally when I'm busy, but it is always there and tiresome to say the least! I hate the area being touched (after all it feels like sunburn!) but it is something you adjust to. There are medications that can help, but a good study of the side effects lets you work out the balance you need and whether it is something you can put up with or if you need to deal with it.

Phantom sensations: OK, so while writing this or talking about my legs or feet, I get them. I feel them not actually as in I can feel them again but I get the sensation of pins and needles every time I try to move them. I still try every now and then or when I am being asked to talk about them in the moment or while writing this, my left calf feels tense, and I have pins and needles in my right foot. Physically feeling my calf, it is totally relaxed and touching my foot – nope, nothing.

Note: All of these change with time and all can be helped without medication which I would explore as soon as you are able to.

I have found having my QL muscle (found in the back) released helps with tightness around my chest and pain. I have also found regular foam rolling or stretching my back and legs really helps. The best forms of both of these, while not always easy is swimming as you really can stretch freely and are weightless. This really helps but do this under supervision and once you have built up confidence in swimming as it can be all rather overwhelming the first time. Something I will come on to later is being self-conscious about being in a chair and also being topless with a large scar.

Summary: Personal perspective – These are all things to look out for in spinal cord injury and things I have to look out for on an almost daily basis. However, pressure sores, headaches, stiffness or numb sensation can all be a precursor or caused by either past injury or you are doing damage without realising it. This can be a bit over the top but you have to find the balance of knowing when you are looking out for yourself then being worried that everything could mean something worse. It is a case of applying common sense, but I would always say there is no stupid question.

If you have had a headache/muzzy head for a few days: Have you checked your skin – the largest organ in human body and you're not seeing anything that stands out? Then yeah, get checked. It might be diet or something else but always seek professional advice from a medical practitioner if it's your GP or consultant. 9/10 it's something simple like forgetting to drink water frequently or missing a meal or pulled a muscle you maybe can't feel yourself. These are all things you come to learn how to spot and the symptoms that follow. With time and asking, what feels like a silly question at the time, can save you a hell of a problem later down the line. There is no need to put yourself at risk should be the main takeaway note – I have done all three and more and have had to be checked.

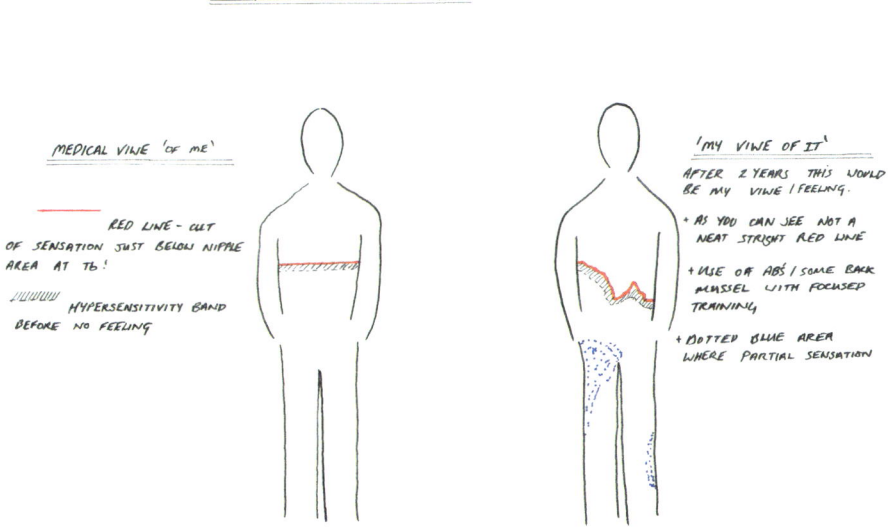

3. CARE BASICS & PRESSURE SORES

Self-care basics: This can be a sensitive topic as we all need to do these things. We just now have to do them in a different way and I guess after having a ton of nurses poke your ass or change your catheter you probably won't blush too much!

So, care basics: Well, what I mean by this is the basic stuff that keeps you from getting into trouble. So, movement, protecting your skin, prep for the worst (yes, carry a backpack). Yeah, it's shit (pun intended) but we have to talk about bowels — and not to take the piss (pun intended again), but yeah, bladder too!

Movement: What do I mean by movement? Well, you'll become what my nan would have called a 'fidget ass', e.g., can't sit still, change from chair to sofa to dining chair and move your legs over. Now and then I rest one foot on top of a knee and then swap over. I sometimes put a cushion either behind my back or sit on it if I am going to be stationary for a long period. I also stretch the upper body twisting from side to side. All these small movements add up to you avoiding **pressure sores. You do not want to get a pressure sore** as they are very annoying and hard to get rid of. Inspecting your skin daily, yes daily is also important — it's the easiest thing to do to avoid getting a pressure sore but if forgotten, it's very hard to get rid of if you get one.

Preparing: So, I have a backpack I carry on the back of my chair, it helps me stay organised (it's actually the one I had on me when I had my accident; I stitched it back up, like me).

It contains cleaning wipes, gloves, lube, catheters, waste bags, sanitary pads, water, meds for spams, paracetamol, small first aid bag, Swiss army knife, radar key, spare pants and I used to carry trousers too – you wouldn't believe how many times these have come in handy!

At first, it's all a balancing act and you don't need to go overboard, but learn your limits and know what you may need. For me, this means if I'm out and about for over 2 hours, I know I'm covered. If something goes wrong, I have the things I need to sort myself 99% of the time and feel fresh and clean at all times. Feeling this way gives me independence throughout the day as the bag is always there and ready to go so, I don't need to worry. I just pick it up and go if I need to pop out.

Bowels: OK, this is something that is mostly going to be impacted by diet and routine which I will go on to later. The rule of thumb is have the bag, wipes, gloves, lube and a spare set of pants (I say pants being a man, but I mean underwear.) and you're set. It doesn't mean you won't ever have an accident, but if you do, then you're covered to deal with it.

Bladder: This is much more of a balancing act and depending on your own bladder you will need to find your own routine and react accordingly.

I personally work on a system of every 3 hours to go for a wee: 9am, 12pm, 3pm, 6pm, etc. I also have three extras, one after I wake up before my coffee, then one hour after the coffee, then also one just before bed. (Which I so elegantly call a 'security piss'.)

I cut drinking any fluids 2 hours before I go to sleep unless I want to wake up in the night and set an alarm or if I'm working thought the night.

The other part of what I do every day is wear a pad (not a diaper(!) or the male version as it bulges and rustles about). But I use four bits of toilet roll folded in half, then have a sanitary towel (yes, i steal from the ladies as one, they work better and two, they are scented) with wings and place it in there to catch any spillage. This keeps everything fresh and has felt more comfortable than male alternatives on the market. While some people may laugh this off and take the Mickey that's fine but hey, I've been caught out only once in nine years!

This happened because I was fixing an engine and leaning over which put pressure on my bladder. The fact I wasn't sitting upright meant the pad shifted, however I had my bag so I could sort myself out. It was no big deal, and no one knew.

They will now but hey, do I care? Nope, not in the slightest! I also learnt from this that it's a good idea to go to the loo before working on engines or putting pressure on your bladder area, e.g., lower abdomen.

Washing (Personal Hygiene): With a lower limb disability especially if you have bladder or bowel issue this is important. Now like everyone even without a lower limb issue, you have to pick shower or bath. Baths are a harder transfer, but they can be better. I love long baths or showers (obviously seated), however, with both, one thing to think of is the main part of the seat has to be padded. Anything you are sitting on should be padded. After trying cushions and an assortment of adaptations that are stupidly overpriced, a solution is simply a folded towel in the bath or on a shower seat to sit on. They grip and are soft enough to allow you to have a good soak.

Note: May be clear to some but don't add soap to the towel as it makes it slippery – I learned that the hard way. (Yes, I did give myself a slap for being a dumb ass.) On both my shower chair – a fold down one and in my bath, all I do is take a regular bath towel and fold it to cover my hips and then place it on the seat dry. Once I have had my shower or bath, I rinse it out. If I shower or bath daily, I wash it once a week. If less frequent, I give it a clean and dry. To me staying clean and washing every day is a mostly frustrating task but feeling fresh and clean in the morning after my breakfast and after using the loo is just a good way to set up my day and is a good habit. Teeth, shave, shit and shower.... set to crack on. I sometimes also bath or shower at night if I have had a workout or just to help relax muscles. The trick is to make the transfer process is as easy and smooth as possible.

Having things in an order of which you use them saves you time and cuts out rushing. I can be washed shaved and out the bath without rushing in 15 minutes. Note – I say this a man with short hair. I did grow it once to raise money for children with leukaemia who needed wigs and I have a huge amount of respect for women with long hair; what a pain it is! But it was for a good cause but added like 20 minutes onto a wash though... urrghh.

SUMMARY OF CARE BASICS

In essence this gives you the outline of what you will build into a routine that will make yourself feel as independent as possible, which after being given the confinement of the chair is what you will want to be.

My little saying/motto, is simple...

> *"Plan for the worst, aim for the best and hope for the happy middle."*

In short, you can be prepared for the worst case, e.g. planned toilet accidents or even injury. You can hope for the best day out and only need to use the water in your bag but if a small accident should occur, you're covered and ready to deal with it.

Personal perspective: This also keeps you fresh and a good steppingstone of routine to follow. In regards to personal hygiene and feeling smart and fresh, I have found this gives you a good start to the day and I find it makes me feel more comfortable and confident.

As I say it is a process and you practice at it. There are many bathroom adaptations that are out there – bars, seats and rails. Two things I have found to be helpful is a hand towel folded on the top of the loo brackets if not a disabled loo as this reduces a risk of injury. If you slip, those brackets are metal. Also grab bars can be handy should your upper body strength not be enough at first. My personal view on bars and bath boards is that while I am strong enough to not use them, it is just a passive exercise (a happy by-product). However, airing on the side of caution, I would use the bars and boards. It takes a while and even I know, one day I will need to use them every time. For now, I'm good but it takes practice. When I did start to transfer i did so with dry bath and trainers and shorts, then things get more interesting when you add water e.g. less balance and certainly needs to be practiced to be able to hold your own weight. As I say, practice and be safe. Personal view.

4. EATING AND DRINKING

These two have the biggest impact on how you can progress smoothly from your old self to your new self. Now it seems like a lot to take on board and what you will have been told so far is to drink more water as things take longer to pass through your system, e.g. food.

To start understanding your eating or diet is the hardest to get your head round, but still doable. In my situation as ever, I knew things would take longer to pass through me and would I become constipated on a regular basis. Why is this? Well at my level T6, your gut is paralysed so naturally everything moves slower. Having to take lactose, fibre supplements drinks and Senokot was just a pain in the back side. (No pun intended.)

Although recommended by the doctors, I cannot be bothered with taking another three medications that I would have to try and take 30 minutes before food, one at night and another straight after food. It was just too complicated for me, so I wrote down my favourite foods and found out what category they landed in such as protein, fibre, carbs, etc. I then worked out the type of meals I could make. Then I spoke to a nutritionist and said, "I am fed up with taking all these medications and yet still having an inconsistent s**t." Yes, I worded it like that. No point beating around the bush or blushing about it! I did say this would be blunt! Luckily however, I formed a diet plan over the course of two months and implemented it, slowly building up an understanding of how my body would react to certain types of food, enabling me to eat more freely.

The one concession I ended up with and had to only really consider was the volume of food.

This was because I didn't want to be a beach ball on wheels and get fat, so my meals are spread out across the day. I eat much earlier in the day than I used to; allowing my gut extra time to process it and letting my body burn off what I ate. After a few years, I know where and how I can push the limits of this 'diet' – for lack of a better term. More or less, I can eat anything I want, and it was very worthwhile understanding this as I haven't needed to take those medications since. So, it's important to remember, if you put in the time to listen to your body and respond to its new needs, you do adapt. Take time in doing this as it is trial and error but it's better to do this than having to be constantly reliant on medication. In my view, this is much less of a headache! This is how I have found it to be, and what works for me is smaller meals earlier in the day, then high fibre towards the end of the day.

Drinking has the next biggest impact on your bladder and gut. So drinking coffee or tea in the morning, as hot drinks help open your gut after only 15–20 minutes. It also helps me personally wake up as I now only take one medication and it makes me very drowsy in the mornings but after a couple of cups of coffee, I'm good to go both for the toilet and get to work.

Breakfast is something protein rich but with a fruit juice; the less sugar the better but if it does have sugar, I make sure to burn that off by doing more movement throughout the day.

The other main drink through the day is water. At the beginning I would I keep a marked bottle which meant I could keep a steady flow of fluid throughout the day. Now it is all second nature, and every 1.5 hours I drink and I know in 1.5 hours I will need the loo. As I have said, in the evening I try to keep fluids to a bear minimum or none at all two hours before bed. But hey, if the evening is good and I want to have a drink with friends or family, I do and I set up a timer for 1.5 hours. Or if I've consumed more than 600ml or two cups or glasses of fluid, then I just set an alarm to get up in the night to go to the loo. It is just that simple. This was learnt by trial and error and I do suggest incontinence sheets for your first few tries. This will become easier and after time and practice this will not be required at all.

Exercise will factor into this later, but the above will help you get a balance and it's important to first get to know the new you! And be prepared for the odd reaction, e.g. if you drink alcohol, milk, warm drinks, they all react differently and you need to learn which one does which. For me, wine speeds things up so certainly set the timer! If a warm drink, consider the loo if in the evening before bed. I have found cold milk to swig before bed just to quench thirst is a safe bet but can alter dreams. This is how it affects me, but a test is also worthwhile especially if you're trying a glass of wine also doubling up as a muscle relaxant!

While I am giving you my own personal view and perspective on it, I would seek professional help with a nutritionist. It is the best advice I got and I think in some ways opened my eyes to how I could keep my independence.

With eating and drinking in my life prior to being on wheels, I would never be worried about over-eating or drinking. When on wheels I was concerned about becoming a beach ball on wheels.

Trust me when I say it's not easy and it isn't the best feeling in the world when you misjudge it, but trial and error at home is a lot easier to deal with than when you surrounded by people and out and about.

Foods

Protein   Carbs   Dairy   Fibre

Protein	Carbs	Dairy	Fibre
Chicken	Bread	Milk	Brown bread
Fish	Pasta	Cheese	Porridge
Egg	Rice	Yoghurt	Bran flakes
Nuts	Cereal		Brown rice
Pork			
Beef			

The above is a very basic list of the main foods I personally eat but a dietitian will be able to expand on it all which will be worth its time and cost.

Summary so far: I have hopefully got you covered on the basics and you are finding this either insightful or useful. I think that you have to be open with the professionals around you and open to suggestion when you first find out you're going to be on wheels. These changes take time to set in and also an important part is not letting anyone (even me!) tell you how you should be feeling. Keep track of your own emotions and also your own body changes as it is different for everybody and unique to the individual.

If you are reading this and you are not the person in a wheelchair or have a spinal cord injury for life, please understand me when I say this will give you insight into the basic fundamentals of the chair/injury or disability. But it is my own personal approach and perspective. It is not a goal or a guide book because everybody copes in their own way and should be free to do so.

When I was first transferred from a general hospital 4 weeks after my accident to a hospital with a Spinal Centre, I didn't want my friends or family visiting or even Googling spinal cord injury. I wanted privacy to deal with it on my own and to get in and out as quickly as possible while learning as much as possible. I didn't like it but I will touch on this later.

Monday
Breakfast – cereal or toast with coffee
Lunch/dinner – main meal high protein chicken or fish
Snack – high fiber

Tuesday
Breakfast – boiled egg/coffee
Lunch/dinner – pasta if early
Snack – brown rice with sauce

Wednesday
Breakfast – toast and coffee
Lunch/dinner – red meat day with pots
Snack – branflakes or porridge

Thursday
Breakfast – bagel toasted with ham
Lunch/dinner – chicken or fish with plain rice or pasta
Snack

Friday
Breakfast – porridge
Lunch/dinner – pork chops and sweet chilly noodles
Snack – cereal bar or homemade flapjack

Saturday
Breakfast – scrambled eggs and brown toast
Lunch/dinner – chilly and rice
Snack – sausage roll

Sunday (the exception)
Breakfast – coffee, bacon and eggs
Lunch/dinner – well it has to be a roast dinner
Snack – nil ... well maybe some chocolate

5. HELP

Asking for help/being offered help are two very different things. Asking for help can be or feel like one of the hardest things to do, but there is absolutely zero shame in it. People seem to find it hard for so many reasons. But feeling shame – I don't believe that should even be on the table. I say this because in my ten years on wheels, I have asked and been given help a lot. I also have had to fight my corner sometimes and realise that what I am asking for isn't unreasonable.

    An example of this would be when I was first on my 'path of understanding my spinal cord injury/disability'. I got to the spinal centre and the head doctor came around and I wanted him to explain it to me in more detail. He just patted me on the shoulder and said, "Just accept it," and walked out the room. I was angry and upset by this but realised what had happened. He thought I wanted a cure and to know how he was going to make it all better. I had to ask him again twice and explain exactly what I wanted to know and why (this would be asking for help and fighting for it). I did this by writing down my questions. When it comes to this type of thing there are no stupid questions and there is no shame in asking for help or seeking professional advice and support. However sometimes, sadly you do have to push for it. To accept something life changing you do need to understand it at a base level and know you probably won't be able to fully understand it all.

Being the cocky little shit I am and can be, I wanted to get the f**k out of the spinal centre as soon as I could, as I hated it. Why? Because from my own viewpoint everyone was miserable, and I found that harder to deal with than my own injury. OK, you're in a chair – adapt, try something different. I just couldn't get my head round it that there were people let's say less worse off than me who were just a misery to be around. And then others who were worse off than me that where just awe-inspiring and made me think, "Well if they are not moaning, what leg do I have to stand on? Crack on." (Yes, I know I have no legs to stand on, but you know what I mean.) Also I wanted to be the person with the quickest record out of there.

I ended up treating it like a job. I took notes in the wellness classes, I went up to the greyest, oldest looking wheelchair users I could find and probably not meaning to, but bluntly, maybe even rudely (without thinking) asked if I could ask some advice with what I thought would be some 'stupid questions'. This was no different to looking in the back of the textbook for a degree, but it also backfired a couple times. Not everyone who is in a chair and is grey has been in it that long, and not everyone in a wheelchair in a spinal centre is there because of a spinal issue, or has the same viewpoint. In some cases it can be also bad advice, as everyone is different, and some people don't really care about their longevity.

What I did learn from the people who kindly gave me their advice and time, was gold dust information about the 'cheats', (the 'hacks' for lack of a better term) the tricks of longevity in a wheelchair and a pattern formed on the most popular concepts, ideas and methods. Yet these are not taught to you by the nurses, physiotherapists, doctors or OTs.

Why? You may ask. Well the answer is sad because it is red tape, and out-dated information and the set of rules that must be followed. Now in the real world, i.e. your life, these are base lines that are good to go by yes, as they are proven methods and safe. But they also are ass-covering red tape drawn up by people who probably have to work within a set system of rules and regulations. (By 'system' I do mean the NHS who did save my life and I do have the utmost respect for.) Yet sadly in the spinal centre and my rehabilitation time, there was, and still is only the set standard of practice which can in my view, limit your perspective on future life and plans. But as you will see, things do get whispered…

I did receive some of the whispered advice from some of the above professionals which was good, but it was also whispered due to it being outside their rules and framework of the NHS.

So, there is a gap in there with the overlay of information and you do have to be careful from where you're getting it from and whom. An example of this is pressure relief to avoid pressure sores. In the classes they tell you to transfer using a sliding board and then lay on one side. They also suggest holding yourself up by taking your bum out of the chair and also not to ever wear jeans. The real-world advice is different. The movement suggested requires two transfers and also a lift that is very hard on the shoulders which you are going to need to keep as healthy for as long as possible. The real-world answer is to become a fidget ass. You need to lean from one side to another giving relief for one side and then do the same on the other side. This takes the pressure off your 'glutes', e.g. bum or buttocks. Also, by using a cushion to sit on at a different angle is a good idea i.e. leaning forward or shifting back. I will draw in some diagrams,

With transfers, a sliding board is good to use once you have the hang of it but you are not always going to have one with you, so here are a couple of tips.

Like checking your brakes! A quick test of this every morning can save you from falling out of a wheelchair. Also, learning how to position the chair as close as possible to what you wish transfer onto or into and should your upper body strength not be strong enough this allows minimum risk and with the correct position, minimum effort. Note: Also if you move your legs halfway into to say a car footwell that's half the job and your body will naturally follow. Just ensure the door handle has slightly bigger bolts which can be done very cheaply with no difference in look should you need them.

Another tip would be always your brakes and if found not be working for whatever reason, put the chair with something solid behind it so you don't fall back. I have had to use my shoes before like car chocks when a break has failed. I again have added diagrams in chapter 28 to show you.

Being offered help: Now if you're still in hospital and it is from a medical person, then yes but see what they are offering first before committing to it and accepting it as the right way or the only way forward. Also think about how this will work in your daily life. There is no reason to feel bad about asking to think about the advice given.

A personal perspective for me was in mapping my seat pressure. I had lost a lot of weight in the 7 weeks after my accident, and I was wanting to get in and out of the spinal centre as quickly as possible. The mapping showed pressure on my hips and bum area to be too high on the left, so they suggested a change in seat which I did. I thought it was not a big deal and that would be good if it takes the pressure off. Now, bear in mind I hadn't had a problem before with my skin or pressure sores, but checking my skin daily I noticed a red patch. After three days of my new cushion I went back and questioned it, and it was the start of a pressure sore. This is not good as it takes ages for skin to recover, so needless to say the new cushion went out the window and my old one was back.

Now this is me noticing change over a period of time. They only had the ability to take a snapshot and recommended the different cushion which was not the best move. Luckily I was on high alert for pressure sores as they mean being stuck for a prolonged period of time while they heal. And that means generally off your chair and yes, on your side which isn't practical.

The other side to being offered help publicly is although it really is nice for someone to offer, you won't always need it. I make it my life mission to say, "I'm good but thanks for offering." 9/10 times because I try to keep myself as independent as possible and there may not always be someone to help me. But being rude to someone offering help may stop them from offering it to someone in the future that does need it or may be too shy to ask! So bear that in mind when you are shopping or in a car park getting your chair out. If you need help then yes, take it but if you don't, be polite. I say this as you will be asked a lot and it does get annoying to be asked all the time.

Another few lines I have used is, *"I'm good thanks. I like to try and keep myself fit,"* with a cheeky wink when putting the shopping in the car. Or when in the gym, with a laugh I say, "Where were you for my first 6 sets! But thanks for offering". Also another is, *"No, I like to make it look difficult,"* with a wink and a thank you.

Swimming has by far been the funniest however, right by the edge and being asked if I need help then say, *"No, I'm good thanks,"* then promptly throwing myself out the chair into the pool. The look on the faces was priceless but I wouldn't advise you try it as I am a bit on the risk-taker side, and I have taken a long time to build up the strength in my upper body and remaining core over the years.

Note: The reason why I say all of these things and the way I do, is simply to put them at ease with a sense of humour to it. Being offered help from a complete stranger is nice, however they don't know your condition or what you actually may need but a happy reply means they will offer again. It can also kill the questions you can get as they don't view you (as disabled or weak) from that point onwards as they can see you are just getting on with your life. Questions you get asked is the next chapter.

Short side story and context in regards to upper body strength and this is just to touch on it as I will write a whole chapter about it. I was injured in October 2012 and was in ICU/general hospital for 4 weeks, then a spinal centre for 6.5 weeks. (Someone did tell me the record was 7 weeks to get out, so I had to beat it!) Time to get back in a gym which was next door to the spinal centre. I had been going there from week two or three of being in the centre. It was five weeks after my accident, and I went to the gym with my dad the first time. I say this because I was at peak fitness when I had my injury, and I wanted my strength back! But I did have 13 broken ribs, so it was against all medical advice to do this.

 I did do one or two sensible (well, which i find sensible) things upon arrival at the spinal centre; I took as little pain medication as possible and by the time I was at the gym I was on only paracetamol for the pain.

 The other small sensible thing I did was take my ego (which seemed to be outrageously large) out the window but this is the best way to test the 'new waters'. It also happens to be the best way forward so the weight I could lift dropped from 40kg per arm before the accident to high repetitions of 10kg, then 8kg, then 5 kg during recovery.

I would also find the path with the hill and push myself up and down that thing as much as I could stand. It was also the second place I burst into tears with my partner five weeks in. I talk about that later.

With every exercise, *I did high repetition but with lower weight or resistance*. I did this as much as possible and over the course of three months. When I was discharged after 6.5 weeks, to my relief my ribs had healed more, and I could push it a bit harder.

This again is not what I would advise as it is my personal approach. I even would go as far as to say from my viewpoint that if I hadn't taken this approach and had that alone time to push myself up and down that hill, sneaked out to the gym in the night, I think psychologically for me I would have gone a bit stir crazy and for me it would have been worse. Physically it probably didn't do any favours to my ribs as they were still broken and healing, so it is just food for thought.

Summary: Asking for it and being offered it as you can see are two very complex fields of which I can really only give my own personal opinions and observations. I have now come to know asking for help isn't wrong or shameful in anyway and also to take my time before just taking the set advice.

In relation to being offered help, as I have explained; yes, you are in the chair, and it can get annoying and repetitive, but I have spoken to people not in chairs that have had such negative experiences when offering help and they never bother again. This to me is not the way you should treat people, as one day you or someone else may need help so be polite you may be helping not just yourself but someone else down the road and manners however tiresome, are free.

FAIR WARNING ON THE NEXT CHAPTER.

OK, SO WHILE EDITING IT IS HAS BEEN SAID THAT IT'S MAYBE BETTER TO LEARN WITHOUT WARNING AND YOU HAVE TO TAKE IT AND DEAL WITH IT AS IT COMES. BUT I PERSONALLY WISH I HAD KNOWN WHAT I WOULD BE ASKED SO AS TO BE PREPARED. SO, READ ON AT YOUR OWN DISCRETION...

6. THE SOMEWHAT STUPID QUESTIONS YOU GET ASKED

I find this probably the hardest part to deal with myself and it can be tricky to navigate through when asked some of the questions below. I do bear in mind it is only natural to ask some of these as I was relatively young at 24–25 in a wheelchair and I suppose you would think, "What happened to him?" (Thought to myself – *why does it even matter?*)

In being asked these questions I found that there is always context to the social situation you are in, but the questions I get most asked and never was warned about being asked were as follows. (I bring this up as this way you are prepared for them – unlike me. So, hopefully it helps.)

The first is when meeting someone new. The first question they ask is, "So how did you end up in that?" followed by a gesture to the chair. Whilst this is a natural thing to be wondering I suppose, I would say I am a little more jokey or blunt depending on the type of person asking me. I have found people who want to know and are polite. They let it naturally trail into the conversation or give me the chance to explain first to just get it out the way. So my response to your first question to me can depend on my mood but sometimes I speed through what happened, shrug my shoulders and that's that. Others I have just point blank refused to answer saying, *"Look I'm* here to clay shoot, not bring up my injury. Let's move onto a different question."

I have flat out lied about what happened to one or two making up silly stories. This is usually when a friend is with me and I see if they bite, but then I do say the truth, but it highlights the question and puts some humour into the situation. Honestly, who wants to explain what is probably something that is a trauma and what does it matter anyway?

Some of the stories I have used are:

- I ordered one of those mattresses off the telly and woke up like it.
- I was in Africa on holiday where I was jumped on by a cheetah like Adam Sandler was.
- I just enjoy it really rough in bed and it went too far.
- I don't actually remember shit. I'm in a chair what the hell!? (I then scream and roll off down the path lol!)
- I did it while playing ping pong.
- I drank too much water one night and something happened
- It was caused by a pigeon flying into my back.
- I fell over with a backpack on. Odd though – it had a pillow in it.
- I'm not actually needing to use the chair; I'm just practicing for a movie role I've been waiting ages for the call back audition though – it's been months!

There have only been very few occasions I haven't even given an explanation and the reason for it is simple, "Well it doesn't really matter, and it isn't your business, I just get on with life."

As I say, it is a natural thing to wonder and ask about. How you respond to the question does set up or shut down the follow-up questions or they realise the first thing they asked is probably the last thing you want to talk about; it being a rather traumatic life event in most cases. However, the follow-up questions and others I still get asked:

- Can you still feel your legs?
- How did that happen?
- Do you miss walking?
- Can you still drive?
- Can you still have sex?
- Can you have children?
- So, do you have a career?
- Can you still work?
- How do you mange in that thing?
- Can you do any ticks in it?
- How do you go to the loo?

Now these are just a few of the many questions I get. Most of them I do tend to answer as I am not too fussed by anyone knowing any of these. But I personally prefer to not be ambushed with the question, i.e. it being the first one out of their mouth. Ask about the weather first, at least! I did nearly get a t-shirt printed in the first year or two saying,

'Motorbike & me vs road and tyre = wheelchair'

Note: In editing this – I do give the elderly people and children more leeway or a "sensible response" as children have what seems to be a innocent curiosity that I wouldn't want them to fear someone in a wheelchair. It is funny as their parents are normally mortified their child has just asked but I always say that it's OK and smile. Older people I find ask bluntly without thinking or any rude intention. Also I partly believe in just giving them a quick response as they probably have less time on the earth than me. (Slight joke in that.)

UNDERSTANDING WHY 'THEY' ASK

After ten years, I have come so the basic conclusion, It is morbid curiosity and understanding of something that isn't seen on a regular basis. I have noticed this happens less the older I get in the wheelchair, but still does happen now. I wasn't ever really warned about these types of questions or how often they come up.

Questions do come up frequently but also so do stupid statements such as:

- So I guess you will be in the Paralympics!
- Do you know this person? He/she is also in a wheelchair.
- Wow, you whizz along in that thing!
- I'm surprised you're still allowed to drive.
- I would hate to be in a wheelchair.
- It's odd seeing someone young in a wheelchair.
  (Sadly, I get less of this now at 36 lol.)
- I'm surprised to see how able you are.

Again these comments are not meant to be hurtful, but they happen, and I always take them all with a pinch of salt and not too seriously because truly there is no need to stress over it. It will only cause you a headache and you don't have to explain or respond if you don't want to.

Another key aspect of this is the questions your family, friends or partner can and do get asked. I have found that they have come to understand not take them too seriously and generally just answer them. But my family, friends, partner can get defensive on my behalf which is why I briefed all of them about it. However, it does still happen, and people will ask or say things such as:

- Bet you have to do a lot for him around the house!
- Must not be easy living with someone with a disability.
- Have you considered moving on?
- How does he stay in shape?
- Do you have to help him get dressed or washed?

I have felt more embarrassed for the people asking these question than I have for myself.

Note: I have realised after ten years, there are four categories of people:

1. Totally unaware of you, they just don't notice.
2. Too friendly, offer help at every chance. They know someone or they have themselves been in a chair for a short while and think they know it all.
3. They're scared if they get too close, they may catch whatever put you in a wheelchair.
4. Lastly, the observers. They watch you like a hawk and see how you do things and are just confused or interested in what they are seeing.

I have formed these categories purely on my personal observation and perspective.

Before I was in chair I believe I would have fallen straight into category number one. Apart from noticing the odd mobility scooter I never really saw or even noticed wheelchair users. Once I was in one however, they were bloody everywhere! It's kind of like when you buy a car then notice the same model everywhere. The same happens with wheelchairs. The term for this is called "frequency illusion" at least that is what I found. I also check out the chair they're in, the make and model, the cushion, wheels, the fit and the look.

7. ADAPTIONS FOR THE HOME AND DAILY LIFE

What I am going to cover is ramps (fixed and portable), kitchen adaptions, bathroom modifications, handy things to have, sofas and beds and some other bits and bobs.

First advice I would give which sounds stupid; know your width i.e. the distance between your wheels and add 3cm or inches either side (the extra distance is so you don't drag your knuckles across the door frame – it hurts). This is so handy if you're going to a new place to know door openings/widths, etc. Ask before you set out.

So I'm 26.5 inches + 2.5 = 29 inches. Metric total is 74 cm rounding up, so this means sometimes I catch my wheel on the frame of the door. (I am in a Ti Lite ZRA light weight wheelchair.)

Ramps: There are two types – fixed and portable. I have a set of lightweight portable ramps which are not covered by the NHS, but they are worth the money as not all buildings are accessible. They generally live in the boot of my car. They don't take up much space and are very handy.

Fixed ramps: I have owned a home and also rented a few. A permanent option is concrete, which is very expensive and also in the winter with ice, it's tricky to say the least. When I have rented, I always just built ramps overly wide but out of decking wood and joists, with shed lining on the top. In the winter this adds grip when salted and then they also can be deconstructed and taken to the next place if you're moving. The only time I have made a concrete ramp was when it was a rather large hill up to my workshop and I also wanted to run cars, bikes or quads up it, but also it was very steep and not a 1:20 gradient which is recommended gradient.

Why are the wood ramps wide? Well, if I have my dog with me or shopping it means I have plenty of space to do a 360 and have a bag or dog next to me. Also the cost is relatively low and if painted and looked after it lasts a good long while.

OK, so outdoor ramps covered…

I have also built internal ramps for my kitchen. I was a chef for ten years before this accident, so the kitchen is my place in a house, much to everyone's pleasure, I think — well, I hope so. I love cooking!

The kitchen: Sides are often too high, and you can get some really cool adaptions for the kitchen that lift up and down with the push of a button. These cost thousands of pounds but are overkill, in my opinion. The next option is the council's solution which is to pay to concrete the floor higher. This is good in theory, but your dishwasher, washing machine and cooker all have to be either relocated or adapted. Also the waiting list is normally rather long and if you're renting it's unlikely that a landlord will agree to this. My fix is some posh decking, so I spoke to a local carpenter and drew up some plans which are below.

All in, it cost me £500 and took 2 days to fit. I always look for a good quick option and this worked well. The floor was even protected, and you could still pull out the dishwasher.

This raised the floor height by four inches or about 13 cm which wasn't too noticeable by people who were using the sink or stove. It meant I could access everything as I would normally and was a smart look as the floor was wood chipboard which looked just like floorboards. Another adaption I have seen but not used is a stainless-steel mirror fitted above the hobs so you can see into every pan. Now however, I dont change the floor height. I needed to at first, but I don't now due to my long arm length and experience over the years of being organised and placing things to make them accessible.

Bathroom: Now this is very much dependent on your upper body strength but something I have found not to be helpful is bath cushions. If you like a long soak in the tub then you need to have padding under your backside – yes, your buttocks, bum, arse! Some of these cushions are absolutely useless. The ones with air and suction pads to stay at the base of the bathtub slide and sometimes pop off. Also when cleaning when you've finished your bath to lean over and pull it off can be really tricky and a big stretch down.

My solution is a simple one, to re-iterate my point in Chapter 3, I use folded towels. They don't slide as much oddly, and I can reposition them in an easy way. Also just before I get out of the bath I ring them out, place them into a plastic bag, get out the bath and then pop them in the washing machine on a rinse and dry.

The other adaptions are bath boards to help with the transfer over – these are helpful but take practice to use them correctly, e.g. not catching your back when you lower in. It is also key as if you're too far forward and there isn't enough room. Ideally you want it placed by the wall so your back can have support, and there's less risk of hitting your head should you fall backwards.

I did use these at first for the best part of 3–5 years but they don't fit every bathtub and balance for me was an issue at the time but with some patience and practice, I started to work out where my balance point is.

Note: Balance point with core muscles. If you have ever driven a manual car (sorry, this is the best example I can think of right now) it is like finding the biting point on a clutch, e.g. too little – no movement, too much – lurch forward. But practice and smooth and steady.

Now not everyone will agree with my next suggestion, but it works – well, worked for me.

I built a wooden box in which I would store my medical supplies and it also worked as a transfer 'plinth' to the bath so I could easily slide into the tub. Also, I had a hand suction grab bar rail by the bath and as it was level the 'plinth', it was a nice and easy transfer.

The last thing is the **toilet seat**. You can get a good one that is padded and looks and works no differently to a standard toilet seat, other than the fact it is padded this means less pressure and less rushing as it is padded.

Another good thing to these bathroom adaptions is that you can keep things tucked away, organised and private. Anyone else using your bathroom can't see the many supplies you will need to keep to hand. For me, this is what they now call my appliances which consists of catheters, wipes, gloves, lube, incontinence sheets (useful for chair cushion if getting out bath or pool) and tie top bags. I just call them my medical supplies as that is what they are but in today's culture and to make it more dignified they say appliances which the lovely people at SIA told me. At first, I did ask if I could order a new blender but no, it is just medical supplies.

Thank you should go to the SIA healthcare group and the lovely people there that will email or call monthly and order my meds and supplies. Special thanks to operators Jill, Nat and Alex.

The living room is all about comfort, but also ties into the bedroom which is making sure what you are sitting on is smooth and comfortable. The sofa and mattress should have no buttons or dimples as this can increase pressure areas. In regards to both, it is also useful to have a cushion or pillow that will elevate your ankles above your hips when reclining or sitting, which will help with ankle swelling.

Handy things: Grabbers are useful when things fall to a place that is out of reach. It's important you buy one with a magnetic end and that you try the grip level first. This is a hit and miss process, but the good thing is they are cheap and when you have found one you're happy with, I would keep one in all main rooms and in your car. You would be surprised how useful this is when something has slipped to the back of the boot or under or behind the sofa!

Gloves with gel or rubber grip in your backpack can be very handy. (No pun intended.) Not only do they keep your hands warm but when it's wet, you can still control the chair. You can buy wheels that have a rubber strip built-in but if you go fast and need to stop, you can get friction burn! Due to friction you would have to wear gloves anyway. My shooting gloves have been best so far as they are thin, warm and have good grip. I have had a few other good ones, which I will show photos of (see Chapter 30, **BACK OF BOOK**.)

How prepared do you want to be? So, I personally have found while most place like Halfords or other cycling shops stock things I need, they may not alway be in stock, so I keep a small kit in the garage and one in the car. This includes tyre filler, WD40, duct tape, a set of Allen keys and also a couple of spare Velcro straps.

In the house, I have a couple of spare tyres and inner tubes, an electric pump as the tyres are over 90psi. Trust me when I say, an electric pump is a godsend. Other useful things are grease for the bearings, spare bearings and a set of spanners.

Summary: These are a few of the things I keep for use. I also have a spare chair I bought second hand which is fitted with off road chunky tyres and wider casters to get over rough terrain. For both chairs I have an attachment called a freewheel. These are not cheap, but they are easy to fit onto the chair. They lift the casters up allowing you even greater freedom, but these all come down to your own personal lifestyle, choices and budget will of course factor into this.

Being in a chair can get pricy if you are not careful, however looking after your chair, giving it a clean and learning how to maintain it can save you a world of issues. Also this helps if a problem does occur, you're set to fix it or have the things you need to have someone help you fix it. You might need help with things like inner tyres which are a real nightmare to place in the tyre without slicing them. I still will go to a bike shop and have them do it as it is a real skill.

8. OTS, PHYSIOS, DOCTORS AND PSYCHOLOGISTS

Four categories of healthcare professionals and there are more but these are the main ones I will focus on.

Doctors: It is important to understand the type of doctor you're seeing in regards to your disability if it is a spinal cord injury or something else that has landed you in a wheelchair. Also, understanding doctors – while they have a framework to work with they are as much an individual as you are, and they have their own methods and practices.

Also, by type of doctor, is it a specialist consultant or your hospital ward doctor or general practitioner. All of these have different roles of which you will learn the difference.

The short cut is – **a specialist consultant** who is top in their field, normally peer reviewed and will have published papers.

Your **ward doctor** is usually training in his field to specialise in the field of study. So they will be studying you and applying what they have learnt from a textbook to the real world.

Lastly is **GPs** – well rounded in medical knowledge. They have to be as they see a vast array of conditions and people. Tip: It can be helpful if you have your specialist consultant draw up a letter and meanings behind your condition specifically and what this means for you. Take this with you when

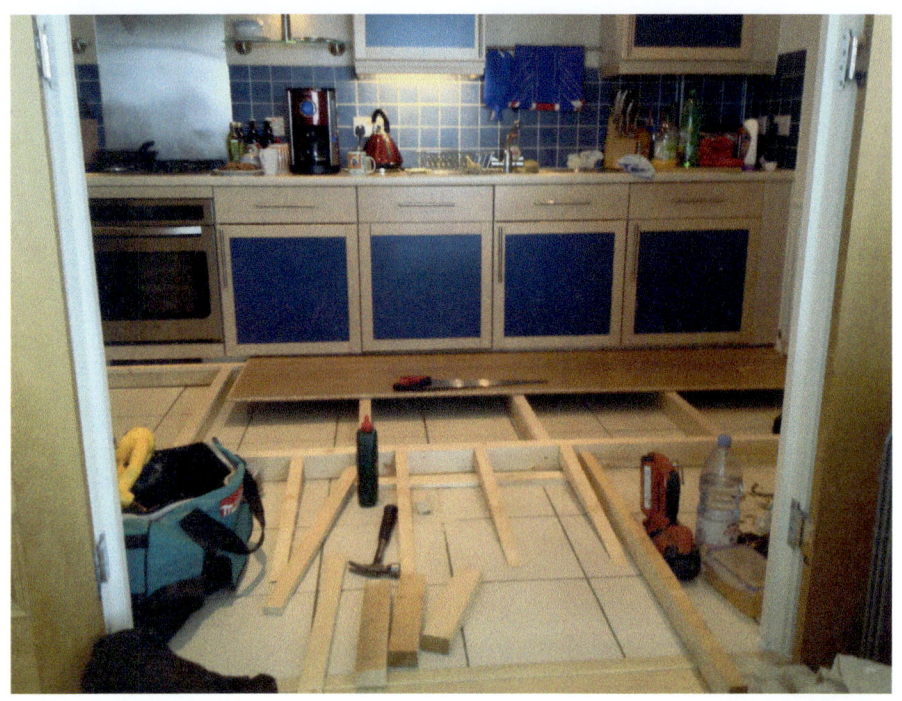
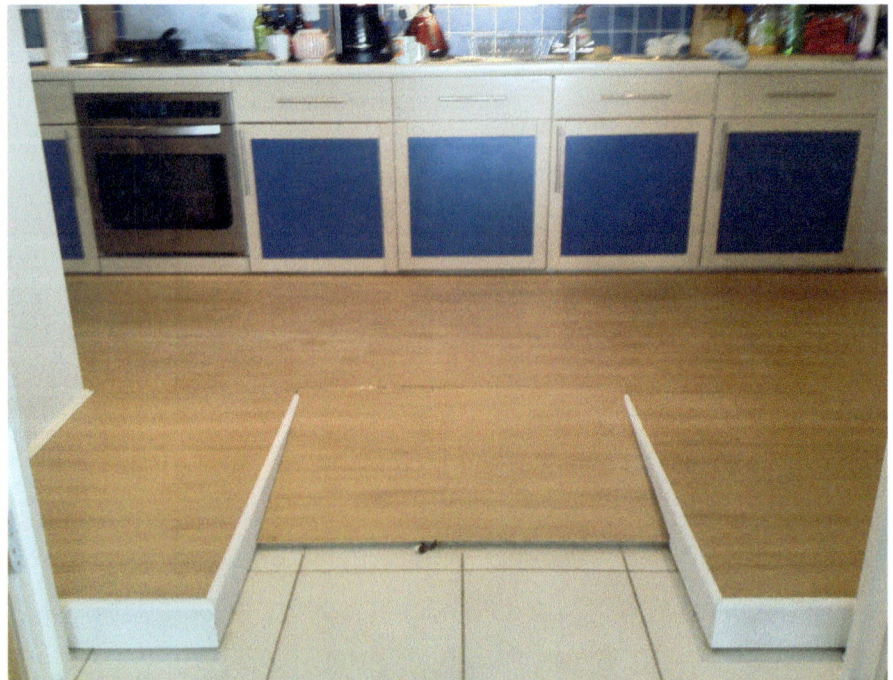

Diagrams I gave to the carpenter for the kitchen are available at the back of the book.

seeing your GP as it can save them time and also be helpful in other ways.

Interacting with GPs: I found that the best doctor I have received care from have been ones I have written to first either via email or letter, asking my questions and not expecting a quick reply. Now for me, I am as blunt as a sledgehammer. I would rather break something up in order to fix it, but in this situation I have to control my own urge to do this and take time, but I still wanted to understand as much as I could, hence the letter of questions. Now some GPs are happy with this while others have flat out refused to engage which I have found to be disappointing, but it also gave me insight into my own needs.

OTs (Occupational Therapists): Well, my personal view on OTs in general is I am sad to say, rather low apart from one OT who worked with me. I have only had them always telling me what I couldn't or shouldn't do and not what I could do or how I could push myself. Their role is very subjective to the individual and to your own personal circumstances and needs. But one saying to me, "I don't think you will ever ride a bike again," to me was a lead balloon approach. So, there is me pulling up videos of people who could ride still and me saying, "And you're recommending my licence be taken away because of this? This chair isn't going to stop me." Well to be fair, she forgot to submit the paperwork and I did get back on a bike but that is a story for another day.

On the whole in the spinal centre, I already had a clear direction in which I wanted to travel. And I would, using my 'sledgehammer' figuratively, smash my past and go through anything or anyone that got in my way. Not being rude but directness and proving not only to myself but others around me, I will just do it and find a way. This was a case of me listening, taking notes and getting the hell out of there. (I still have that notebook and I treated it all like a job.)

Another example of this is trial and error. Going up and down steps or curbs – yep, trial and error but with elbow pads, helmet and knee pads. I must have fallen out of the chair a good few times off curbs and steps but after a couple of days I learnt to understand the tipping point[1] of the chair and how to use which makes life easier. Now falling out is never pleasant but learning how to fall and pick yourself up again is a good idea. You don't want to be going backwards as you will hit your head and if you do start to go backwards, learning how to twist to the side letting the chair take the brunt of the fall is a good idea. You don't want to fall forwards or backwards as that means hitting your head or snapping your wrists which i can tell you hurts. So, if you can lessen that risk by practice even starting by falling on to something soft, it is time well spent.

Psychologists: People to talk to. Yes, it really is that simple but if you don't want to, then don't. Adapting to your new life is tricky and can be very time consuming and emotionally tough on you and family which I will talk about later. But in regards to yourself having an emotional check-up through the first two years, it can be of benefit. At first, I was told to go as I was apparently 'coping too well' but I did go. It was what I thought more or less, but a helpful point was made which I do remember which was – there's no harm in having your car checked before a long trip is there?

---

1 Tipping point or back wheel balancing is the act of controlling the chair on just its two large wheels being able to move forwards and backwards also up and down curbs.

It also hit me later on that getting that check-up is of benefit to not only yourself but to others around you.

Emotional well-being: I personally did see a psychologist later on about year and half after being in the spinal centre. My perceptions of the world changed, my body had stabilised, and I didn't feel as if I was performing at my maximum level in regards to work and happiness. I felt I wasn't doing a good enough job. So I spoke to someone and getting a different point of view was helpful to me. It also shed light on areas I hadn't even thought of which was good for me. But also the person not being personally connected to me or fully knowing me was interesting to see how I was perceived by someone new. It allowed me to be able to express/vent/moan without the feeling of being a burden.

I have saved the best till last, **physiotherapists** – I had one amazing one in my spinal centre. Now they are brilliant in movement and finding out range of what you can and maybe cannot do for now. Mine certainly would push me but in the best way; explaining how it would not only be to my benefit in the long run from a physical perspective, but also how keeping active and fit would have an impact on my emotional well-being. She had amazing insight and was very helpful there and would also advocate on my behalf.

Now I didn't just have one physio. There are two others who had just finished qualifying but they were sadly maybe still learning. I wanted to try FES (functional electrical stimulation) this is where pads are connected to your legs and a small current is applied and the muscles move. This is done while movement of the leg is in motion. This stimulation slows or can even reverse muscle atrophy. The young man in question wouldn't even allow the test for it. I was upset as my legs thinning wasn't something I wanted. Long story short, a slapdash test did get done but results were minimal. The smug look I got from the young physio was unfortunate. Now when I got out the spinal centre and being the sceptic I am, I booked an FES test with a company that ran the machines. Lo and behold, with the right adjustment there was full muscle movement, but this was six months later however, and I had worked out that if my legs remained large, my upper body would have to lug round that extra weight and with the right jeans or trousers you wouldn't notice my legs. I was very self-conscious about this. Now I wear shorts and don't care at all, but this took a lot of time.

The other was again a younger physio woman who just didn't really seem to care about people – she just wanted you to do as she said without explaining why. I did have a run in with her. I said, "I know this is going to knacker my wrists so no thanks." She tried to bait me, so I bit back (smash it approach). Now this wasn't right of me – I tend to be able to cut people down a little too easily, but you sometimes have to just stand up for yourself (well let's now say 'stick up' for yourself) but while being respectful. The minute you swear, you lose any foundation of creditability in your argument.

Whispers: I had them from all of the above, mostly my nice physiotherapist and some from the ward doctors, but remember they do have to stay within the framework or system they are given to protect you and themselves, but they do happen. The two I did listen to had strong connections to wheelchair users, e.g. first-hand experience. I won't go further as I would not want to get anyone into trouble but if you ever do read my book thank you, you saved me!

Summary: This is my understanding of all the medical professionals above from a personal perspective. I do keep saying that as it is a rough guide, but I didn't know about any of this until I was discharged from the hospital spinal centre – e.g. too late!

I will also say yes, i have painted what may seem a dim view and this isn't everyone's opinion, and some will strongly disagree and perhaps rightly so. My perception and opinions are very blunt and to the point and I do tend to rub people up the wrong way some of the time. I can also word things poorly which comes from many years of being a very stubborn chef and I also had to remember the only person you can count on is yourself, even before my injury.

On a positive note – the spinal unit had some brilliant people in there and a wealth of knowledge. The key thing I learnt was to dig for it and ask the questions and set a pace I felt comfortable with.

9. IMPACT ON FAMILY AND FRIENDS

Wow, OK this is going to be the harder chapter to write as I can only give you my observations and my character is undoubtably going to be different from yours. (Probably a good thing.)

Nevertheless I noticed that maybe not just for myself but at the spinal centre and speaking to other wheelchair users even of different kinds of disabilities not just spinal cord injury like mine, it was harder for family, friends and partners to accept. Now this isn't a blanket case. Sometimes it was the other way round and you would have the family unit or friends or partner almost dragging the wheelchair user along emotionally even sometimes physically to help them, but I will try and break this down.

I think I will do this in three ways, so it makes some sense, which I hope it does.

My own personal perspective – OK, as I said before I had my cry with my dad on day one and five/six weeks later when at the spinal centre I had a cry with my partner. I was trying to push her away; it didn't work but the thought got stuck in my head that I couldn't make her happy anymore and I didn't want her inconvenienced by or with my injury. As I've said earlier, I hadn't allowed anyone to see me at the spinal centre without calling first and then only giving them a very small window. I was there to get a job done – learn, work, complete.

I also didn't want anyone knowing my business, like what spinal cord injury really means to you. I forbade my mother and father to go to a lecture on spinal injury. My mother listened and didn't go but my father (being a stubborn ass like me, I guess) went. He did say that it was pointless anyway as he said respect for a person using a wheelchair is one thing but understanding the issues can vary so vastly from person to person. On top of that, you then have the people that are all set differently emotionally. The lecture didn't do what I am aiming for in this book.

In regards to **my partner**, I loved her, and I just felt she would want a normal life and to be as I would say, not troubled by my issues now ten years later we are still together. Was I wrong or right? Well, I think the offer of an 'out' there and then and with time to think, it was still the right thing to do but I am a very independent, stubborn person by nature, and I certainly didn't want her becoming my caregiver or me to be reliant on her.

As I say I blocked most of people that wanted to visit as I didn't want them to see me, and I didn't want to see them. I wanted to have singular focus on the main issue. I did also ask everyone not to Google spinal cord injury and its meaning, but I do suppose it's like a sign that says, "Wet paint. Do not touch." Hahaha, we all know 9/10 what happens then – that doesn't look wet but yes, it is.

Upon reflection ten years later, was this the right thing? Yes, but only because of my own personality and the methodology I use to approach problems.

My friends – This was an interesting dynamic; it would be safe to say I had four that I wanted to see and the others that sent a text to and called. I think it came down to my respect for them and trust in them that they wouldn't cross the line but also allow me to socially engage. Also it allowed me to know the truth. What did they think to the conversation and the way I was dressed and what they thought on certain issues I had or what I would call different social dynamics and approaches. To me, these are friends I trust to tell me as it is the truth unfiltered and clear as day, as that is what I ask for out of my friendships; brutal honesty regardless of feelings. This does work both ways although some don't like it that much, but they know me enough to know I am blunt, truthful and I don't mean things with intended malice.

In regards to my **grandparents** – Being the older generation I would imagine there were questions asked but not to me. I do remember my grandfather saying, "I really hate seeing you in that thing," referring to the chair. He didn't mean this in a hurtful way and knowing him, I wasn't hurt so I jokingly said, "Well I'll jump on the sofa then." He understood the reference and we had a chat about the rugby. They always kept it light around me. I know they had been very shocked though. I always was up to something stupid, so I guess for my family and people that knew me yes, it was a shock and perhaps they thought it was only a matter of time before something happened. They knew me well and with a 'you can't change the past' and just move forward approach, they knew it wouldn't hold me back too much.

General view of others in chairs – Now these are my own experiences. I have seen some that give up or have a low where they close down themselves and their families and friends visit who try so hard to cheer them up yet seem to fail. The moment they leave, the person would break down into tears. I spoke to a few of these people. There isn't much privacy in a hospital. I would say simply, "Want me to go grab a cuppa or a coffee?" Most of the time with passing sobs they would say yes, and I would give them some space and privacy to have their moment, taking just that little bit longer to get the tea or coffee. By the time, I came back they would either sit/lay there, say "Cheers" and/or either we would sit in comfortable silence, or I would let them sound it out of me or just chat.

I would often be asked how I stayed so upbeat with it and how I wouldn't take the negative in. I would say, "Well I guess it's just a process and you have to take it at your own speed but if you wanna talk, we can or just chill."

I did find putting on a comedy TV show even just as background noise and talking about a fun subject helpful – not just for them but for me too to take me out of my own moment. I still do this but now to focus as background noise as I work or a new thing to try to do or adapt to.

I do think speed is a subjective term. There is not really a slow or fast. People say I went fast through both stages of hospitalisation and rehabilitation. Others could turn around and say that maybe taking ten years to finally open up and write down these thoughts has been my true speed. It all depends on what scale or metric you are using. It is just getting back into 'normal life' if there is such a thing!

Being emotionally able to talk openly about it all – is it another goal to get driving again or back on a bike, back to work, travelling or something which I haven't thought of or even reached yet? I would say it is very much a moving scale. I think there are some set goals yes, but I think life in general is ever-moving, changing and only you can see this. The goals change and your plans shift. You change, some things change, and you have to completely scrap others all together. I suppose it is just learning to not beat yourself up and move forwards and onwards and never to get stuck in place unless that is your where you have found yourself to be happy – disability or not really.

Some thoughts from my family:

MY MOTHER'S THOUGHTS

Shocked. Broken-hearted. Sorrow.

I was in Vietnam, and I got a call to tell me that my son had been involved in a serious accident with life-changing injuries. How did I feel? All of the above!

I don't really remember the journey back home, but I did it and went straight to the hospital. When I saw him lying in bed, the stark fact that he would never be able to walk again didn't seem real – he was poorly in bed, that was my thought. But when I saw him being transferred by a hoist into a wheelchair, reality hit. It hurt bad. A torrent of emotions I'd never felt before lasted for several months. I felt overwhelmed by sorrow that this had happened to my boy.

Guilty. Amazed. Frustrated. Acceptance.

These were my feelings on the journey I was on with my son. Why wasn't it me that had sustained these injuries? He was too young for all this. As time passed, I watched his amazing, truly inspiring inner strength grow which I found mind-blowing. My brave, strong, courageous son dug deep and just got on with it; so, I did as well. He'd always been head-strong, and can I say, stubborn? I really don't know where he gets that from! I was his mum and I so very much wanted to look after him and take care of him. I couldn't make it all better. As terribly hard as it was, I had to step back, let him find his own way and keep his valued independence despite all these 'mum instincts'. It's about letting go, respecting and trusting your child, I think.

What led me to the acceptance stage? I'd spoken with a specialist counsellor at the spinal centre in the early days which helped sort my head out a little. And in time, I realised feeling sorrow and sadness about what had happened really wasn't helping in any way whatsoever. But perhaps more significantly, it was seeing Alexandar coping so incredibly well. He does it his way. And he still does.

I find it interesting that some people ask me even now in an upbeat manner how my other son is and then go on to ask in a somewhat sorrowful tone, "And how is Alexandar coping?" I'm puzzled as to their perception of his situation. He takes up and rises to challenges, overcomes all difficulties, still causes me stress and worry (don't all kids?) and I couldn't feel prouder of him!

MY FATHER'S THOUGHTS

How do you as a parent react when you get a phone call saying that it is the hospital and that you need to get down here as soon as possible as your son has had a motor bike accident and a serious injury to his back?

Well because my son has always been a joker, I told the voice to stop messing around. When I realised he was being serious my next question was, "Is he going to die?"

After being told that it wasn't life threatening my next reaction was to kick my office wall hard and call my son a bloody idiot. (I thought that he had been speeding. I was wrong).

I don't remember driving the next ten miles other than bawling my eyes out all the way to collect my wife who then drove us to the hospital. I don't remember the journey; it's all clouded.

On arrival at the hospital we were taken into a small room (my heart sank as I thought it meant that they were going to say he is dead) but instead it was to explain that Alexandar would never walk again. His spinal cord had been snapped.

I cannot explain the feeling of seeing your son lying there strapped up unable to feel his legs other than as a parent, I would say that it felt like being kicked in the balls very hard, feeling sick and not knowing what to do, wanting to take the pain away from him yet knowing there is nothing you can do. Yet his first words (I am choking up writing this) were, "Dad it's not your fault; I would have got the bike anyway."

From then on it was weeks in hospital watching my son be so positive and amazing at the way he handled things – often not the way he was being shown (no change there) and has continued that way ever since. One lesson to learn early on is that although his legs were shot, he was still Alexandar – still bolshy, positive, arrogant, cheeky and determined. The accident didn't change him, only the way he gets around. He is not a disabled person, he is Alexandar. (Just happens to be a wheelchair user.)

Not knowing what would happen, all the questions; you feel you are in a fog. As a parent you want to help in every way possible but not realising how your son is feeling and that he doesn't want you to fanny around him and know all the personal stuff that would be involved for him. Hindsight is a wonderful thing and I now know why he didn't want me to attend a seminar at the hospital all about these issues. **However, it takes time to start thinking straight** as you are in a complete fog and worry for your son/daughter. The daft thing is, my worry didn't help him one bit; he was getting on with life and doing his utmost to get on and get out... I never heard him complain once.

Talking about worrying, on an early visit to the gym with Alexandar he decided to do pull ups (with wheelchair still attached) but got very annoyed with me when he was doing bench lifts with dumbbells when I grabbed one of them panicking he was going to drop it... Oops, my mistake. **As time goes on you learn, try to see things from their perspective** (we should do that for them anyway).

Another lesson from that incident at the gym is to let your son/daughter know that if they want you to help, then they must ask you. After that, don't keep on trying to help or asking if they need help.

Alexandar has got on with life in his determined way. He is still trying to beat me at shooting...ha ha. Nothing is impossible and he has not changed as a person one bit. When I see him, I don't see the chair – I see him as my son but that has been made easier for me by the fact that he has always been so positive. I don't think that you will ever get over wanting to swap places with your child and make things better (that's natural) **but when your son/daughter has moved on with it, why shouldn't you**? Ten years on, Alexandar is still his old self and has achieved lots with more to come. Your son/daughter/partner can do the same and so can you.

MY BROTHER'S THOUGHTS

I was in Lyon, France studying on a year abroad when I received a call from my dad informing me that my brother had been in a very serious car accident. The first thing I needed to know was if he was conscious and if he was OK. Dad assured me he was but that he didn't know much more. Having moved abroad and with our mum being in Vietnam, I felt removed from the situation and quite helpless. It's hard to know what to think in situations of extreme emotion. On reflection, I was worried and scared for my brother's health and life and scared for how my mum and dad would take this difficult news.

Immediately I began looking at flights back to England. I sat through lectures and still attempted to socialise. Luckily for me, I had made some very close friends very quickly that I could share this news with, and they supported me through this. As I awaited news to drip feed from dad, I felt sorry for him that he was constantly updating everyone. I knew my mum would be on her way on the first flight regardless of what Alex said, but I wanted to speak to him first before booking a flight. After speaking with him, he had strict instructions. "Do not come home." Alex has always fought for what's best for me as a person and has always been open and honest with me. If he wanted me to come back, he would have told me explicitly. I did speak to him 2–3 times and each time this point was raised vehemently. We agreed that I would come back at Christmas and visit him in the spinal centre. We stayed in touch throughout and as a brother and a friend, I was sad to not see him. However, I knew that he would prefer it if I wasn't there.

It soon became quite routine speaking to Alex, and not all conversations were about his hospital experience. As the days got shorter and the time to come back to England for Christmas loomed, we planned a visit that I would come and see him at the hospital. I wasn't sure what to think, I was excited to see my brother. When I did see him, he was exactly as he was before the accident, just now he was in a wheelchair. This didn't make me feel any great emotion and certainly wasn't sad or embarrassed because of how well he looked compared to the images and scans he had sent me. I know my brother and his 'crack on' attitude. I wasn't sure of the etiquette of offering to help with things, transfers, etc. I soon learnt if he needed me to do something, he would tell me. I cannot get over how well Alex has taken to being in a wheelchair. I am so proud every day of the challenges he faces and shrugs off and his ability to thrive in whatever he is doing.

10. MAKING YOUR SCHEDULE

This can seem just really overwhelming at first, but it will become second nature in the end and save you so much time and this is something they don't teach you.

I will start by explaining something first but quickly, as this isn't my life story but so you understand, I was a chef for ten years and then I wanted to go back to school and go to university to study architecture. It was a big jump; total career change yes, hard yes, really hard. How did I do this?

I adapted some of the things I learnt while being a chef to uni and scheduling was key in uni. I adapted even further. I liked having money and free time. How did I do it? I had a job in the evenings 9pm–3am at the post office as a chef (term used loosely) and then uni 9am–4pm Monday to Friday, sleep for four and a half hours, 3:30am–8am and then 5pm till 8:30pm

I would stay on campus at university – lectures or not and separate my home life. Any hours out of 9am–4pm was uni work so I never had to do course work at weekends, and I never missed a project which was due to a high level of structure. Other students would always ask me how I would do it, e.g. never work at weekends. I'd say, "Well, I treat it like a job." I don't think anyone really did get that or understand how I could miss out on going out on a Thursday or Tuesday night when the party was on, and I was either in the libary or at work Monday to Friday and very strict with myself. As in cheffing 'fail to prepare,

prepare to fail'. Things can be learnt through failure but let's learn through failure in a way that say, isn't packing your own parachute!

Schedule – How does it help? What are its down sides? So to me the sense of order and structure is key in my world and became second nature. At first I hated it; feeling boxed in at a point. However this passes, as with scheduling and structure, you learn what you need to put in and what you can take out and given your level of commitment to it, the quicker you learn what works and what doesn't. What did I keep track of?

Drinking – time, what type, what volume.

Eating – time, what food group, meal size.

Toilet – time, type, good/ok/bad, if bad how.

Movement – type, e.g. pressure relief, transfer, exercise, getting something and time taken.

Work or task – type, e.g. cooking bins sweep floor, working on schedule time.

Leisure time – type e.g. sitting/laying movie or painting or drawing or playing with dog time spent.

Sleeping – tracking it good/ok/bad type times.

Noting these seven key things is a tedious task but from this you can form a schedule that is most beneficial to you and your new needs or wants. It also allows greater insight should something go wrong. For example, who remembers what they ate say three days beforehand or where they were and at what time.

This is a very intense process but as I say, worth its weight in gold! By forming a base to build upon, then with that base and time, you can alter it to be more flexible and know where you can change or get around things; what your body is saying yes to and what makes you happy.

Given even more time you will find you don't need the schedule anymore and this becomes like breathing – second nature and you run on autopilot, unconsciously doing things at the time you need to do them. An expanse of my formed schedule below:

0600	H^2O
0630	Loo
0640	**Coffee/write a to do list**
0730	Loo
0800	H^2O/breakfast
0900	Loo
0910	Work out
0950	Wash
1000	Loo
1010	H^2O
13/1400	Lunch dinner/H^2O
1500	Loo
1630	H^2O
1700	Relax time
1730	Loo
1800	H^2O/snack

1900	Move and then TV
2000	Loo and rest last H^2O
2100	Prep for bed, loo
2130	Slight drink as in bed meds/loo

This was developed over time and yes, mistakes were made when I started but this is how it ended up to this day if I was to map it out.

Summary: Why in my opinion, is this vital? Well you get to change and adapt so much quicker, and should something go wrong you can pinpoint how and why. Nine times out of ten this can also be helpful when you note a change in health or your emotions or routine in general. But as I say, make your own schedule, take your time in doing so and see just how much you can still do and what new things you can also do.

11. LEARNING YOUR ENERGY LEVELS

Understanding your energy levels. This component is very important, but also only by testing your limits can you work out where/when you fatigue and where you have energy. Understanding this is helpful also when scheduling.

So let's say you decide to do a workout – then you need to know the impact this will have you later on. How do we determine this? Well yes again, by trial and error and starting small, like I pushed up and down that hill at the spinal centre. I learned.

What I learned was also through my diary. It would show me the impact on the drinking levels, what I would need to eat after or before, and the impact it would have on toilet needs, also the movement the day after and how it would affect my sleep. This is the base understanding of doing x activity would result in y outcome meaning z needs to me implemented and this is the trick to learning it. Reaction to doing something is good but knowing beforehand, e.g. being prepared and not just having to react is better.

This is the physical side of it. Now what we haven't talked about is how your emotional levels can have a huge impact on your physical side. This can be fairly difficult and seeing a physiologist to help you navigate these waters will offer much better insight then me – this would be my key advice on it to understanding it.

My own insight into this is some days you just have to rest your brain and body recharge. I do this by keeping off social media and just focussing on something like a book or fixing one of my old bikes or simply writing my thoughts down. The other is watching a really good run of films and having a 'cheeky takeaway', as my brother would coin it.

This for me, is a rest. There are things or times I do make for myself to do the things I enjoy. Luckily, mostly of them revolve around work anyway so I do try and take myself out of my 'work mode' and into something new. It could be a new form of painting, drawing, photography, writing or reading a really challenging book, but this is a life that has been constructed carefully over the last ten years.

The flip side of this is when I find myself bursting with energy. I will have days where I want and need to be as productive as possible, or I want to just have one day to do something that will really be exciting or nuts. This includes for me – going flying or go-karting or a track day to a massively impossible to do list of stuff around the house, giving myself a tick for each one.

Sorry about that. Back to energy levels and the physical side of it. While the ups can usually be explained a little easier either good nights deep sleep or I'm in a really good mood. The other is the drain the day you wake up and you just know it's not going to be a good one on how you are feeling physically.

Drained feeling can be because of the day before or if it is drained with a slightly elevated temperature or chill, this can be a sneaky way of your body saying something is not right. I have had this twice. First time, I woke up in a cold sweat but feeling so sore all over. I was thinking whether this is the flu or a cold, which I would rarely get. I got a warm drink after a shower that seemed to drain even more energy and took forever. The next day I still couldn't get comfortable, but I noticed something – however much I drank, my pee wasn't the right colour and smelt different. Now I do understand how gross this sounds but from that I almost knew it was a UTI (urinary tract infection). When in the spinal centre I had a few but this was the first away I'd got at home. I looked in my book; I didn't go to the doctor, but I had a system flush to flush out the system. Being me, the flush out is a high level of vitamin C, tons more water and soup, lots of soup. UTIs are not pleasant though and you go for the loo like a racehorse but this system flush has worked for me. Also in my case, I have allergies to most of the antibiotics they would prescribe anyway so I do my own system flush. The key is to tune in to yourself but not let it run your life or get too far before seeking medical help. Calling 111 or your GP can be very useful in this situation, but I would advise anyone – if in any doubt, don't take risks, just ring the doctor.

Another drain time that I have had a known cause for physically is sleeping in a stupid position. So I can't move my legs but somehow I must have twisted in the night, and they were over the side of the bed all night. I looked like I had elephant feet! Ha-ha. I also felt so drained and annoyed at how the goodness they had ended up like that. I don't know but that was it; feet had to be up for most of the day to allow blood to be in the right places. Feet swelling is common when you are a wheelchair user because you are not designed to sit down all day! Note – Standing using a standing frame on a regular basis helps blood pressure, heart and slow the bones from becoming weak due to not load bearing.

Headache and energy – There is one other side to having a lot of energy. But a headache, again in my personal experience, like this is from injury. One was simple I had been taking the dog for his walkies and rolls and the little git pulled me into a big metal bollard. Me not noticing at the time because of the big clang of the wheelchair, my toe unknowingly took the brunt. Now it wasn't till I was having lunch an hour later and I just could not settle. I also had a mild headache. Water was good and I didn't feel tired, in fact the opposite. I was very restless. By chance, I looked down and noticed that one of my shoes laces looked tighter than the other. I thought it was odd, so I went to correct it by taking off my shoe. The reason was very apparent. My big toe was huge and my foot was swollen. So, this was a trip to A & E. An X-ray later – yep, that was a broken toe and damage to tendon. I did make the joke about the fact it didn't hurt. Also when the nurse touch it I said, "Ouch," which made her jump and laugh and said, "You prat. Got me!" It was a silly situation to be in, but I also wanted to lighten the mood. I had to wear a boot for a few weeks, take Ibuprofen to keep the swelling down and Paracetamol for the headache. That was the first warning story. The second which I will speak about later, was also a little more of a warning story.

OK, just to note, even I get it very, very wrong sometimes. Below is an example of just how easy it is and how stupid I probably was... Just saying – this is not advice at all.

Again headache and I couldn't sit still. Just had a lovely lasagne I had warmed up from cooking a big batch. Now I had microwaved it and felt the bottom of the bowl which was warm but not hot. I placed it on my lap, rolled to the living room and moved on to the sofa. Not a big deal, right!? Well, long story short, after eating, I couldn't sit still. I thought this was annoying and I started to get a headache. I got up to take a Paracetamol but thought maybe I just need the loo. So I popped into the loo, pulled down my jeans and my – it was clear why I felt like this... Both legs; massive blisters. I almost was in shock. How the hell did that bowl burn me? It wasn't even warm. I'd checked it as I always did after having been warned about people doing this and being an ex-chef, I knew I didn't want 2nd degree burns but yep, I got caught out! So, I had microwaved the bowl, felt it and placed it on my lap but what I didn't take into account was that the bowl was still getting warmer... straight into my legs which I couldn't feel. Yes, A & E again – no joke this time as I was just angry with myself. Now they did give me instructions on what to do and to go back once the blisters had ruptured. The main thing was to keep the area sterilised as infection can easily set into burns. By this point I had a full medical bag at home, and I didn't want to go back again to the hospital (they are somewhat or a sore point for me).

DO NOT DO THIS: I got home that night and ruptured the blisters as I didn't want the agro of it happening in the day and ruining whatever I was wearing. So probably stupidly, I did this wearing gloves, sitting on incontinence sheets. I then tidied up the area cleaned the legs with saline and cut off the blisters with a scalpel, applied an iodine mesh big bandage and wrapped the top half of my legs up. I secured this with duct tape so it wouldn't move in the night. Midway through, my partner asked me what I was doing in our bed kind of just sitting on an incontinence sheet. I had put another on top at this point as there was the blister skin, a little blood and yeah, all the tools where hidden, ha! I said I didn't want to go back for something I could just sort out. Now lifting the incontinence sheet, she went a little pale and said, "Is that effing duct tape? Oh for goodness sake." Long story short, I was careful I didn't get an infection, but I have been trained in this type of issue, so DO NOT TRY THIS. But also, don't take warm/hot bowls on your lap. I ordered a meal tray the next day and it's not happened since.

Energy levels and recognising them as you can tell, can inform you of two things – you having a good day or going to be a bad one. It's the first noticeable thing after you have got up and had your tea or coffee. It's a good indicator as to how you can let your day play out, e.g. by taking it easy or normal plan or having an issue or illness setting in or just had a really good night's sleep and you want to crack on with a lot of tasks or push yourself.

Summary: This is just how my own energy levels seem to present. Undoubtedly these will be different from yours. What won't be different is the fact you can track them, become in tune with them and also start to learn for yourself what they could mean for you. This again isn't something I was taught. I believe this to because everybody is so different, and writing this, even I know what is applicable to me may not be at all to you. It all depends on you and your strategy you wish to take, the path you want to travel and knowing there are options out there for you. Mine? Your own ? And countless others you can take from, but the main takeaway is that you feel happy and as healthy as possible and in control as much as possible regardless of the advice you chose to take.

12. THE PERKS OF THE CHAIR

Yes, the perks. There are some. Due to the nature of this book, so far I figured to move these chapters round as it's not all structure and management of yourself there are some perks. Now you're probably thinking I've at this point lost the plot as to what could I possibly mean. Well let me explain – I don't mean just free parking. ;)

Tickets to movies, shows, places, e.g. entry to concerts, stately homes, F1, Alton Towers; most of these are discounted or your 'carer' for that day goes free. I went to F1 Monza with my dad, and we got to sit almost on the start line, drive into the centre of the track and the ticket for me was nil and dad only had to pay a general entry fee which was 32 euros! Very much worth the 14-hour drive.

Cars – If you're in a position to buy a new one, no vat is payable or road tax. Every three years or if you are eligible you can use the Motability Scheme. Dependent on the car you choose, there could be nothing to pay although they do take the Motability allowance from your DLA or PIP, but you have to only put fuel or electric in the car.

If you hate waiting, you normally find that you can jump the queue or get ushered forward at **theme parks** – this is most noticeable.

In regards to **parking**, if you have that blue badge, then you generally have easy free parking. For me, I normally however just pick a corner spot but it's handy if you're having an off day.

Also handy if you need to nip in somewhere, you can park up on double yellows for a short period. However, do read the advice as it isn't something to make a habit of or abuse.

Hotels are an interesting one as I have found not using or booking through websites is useful. Giving them a ring helps. Just explaining I am in a wheelchair and asking what they can do, as the websites do not guarantee as disabled friendly room. Also you may not want to have a disabled room if you can check them out. (I will talk more about this in travel.)

Travel tickets such as bus, coach and train are discounted. The area you sit in is normally by or near the loo. I do transfer over to a normal seat where possible, but this depends on the seat, e.g. hard or soft and also how I'm feeling.

You also save a ton on shoes!

Another is the **radar key**. These are for accessing disabled only loos. These are handy as they are mostly all set up for chairs. There have been the odd one or two which are a bit untidy but only someone with a radar key can enter. If you forget to take yours with you, it is normally kept at a reception or the shop nearest to the loo.

Access to areas that are not also normally open — I have found this to be a perk for concerts and gigs.

Dependent upon how sociable you are or start to become, there are many **groups** you can join that do either group sport activities or days out. These are normally either very low cost or even free.

There are some **grants** also available to do certain types of things but also in further education there is a lot more support offered.

The last perk is regarding **medical care**. You are buzzed through the line so normally you are seen quicker and treated faster. Yes, this is because you are disabled but it is also good as who likes waiting.

Building a new home – That has some big advantages with the VAT system currently in place, especially if you are designing your home around your chair or your disability.

You can also call the local council refuse and recycling department to inform them you are disabled, and you need your **bins** picked up closer to your door. This is very helpful when you have a long driveway.

Also **council tax reduction** if applicable, is another perk.

If you inform your service providers, e.g. energy, water, internet and/or phone company that you are disabled, they do have in most cases a **quick response team** that will come out with a portable generator or even heating fans should there be a problem with your supply. Or they offer a fast-track fix service normally listed as a 'priority service'.

Also any adaptions or imported goods for use for a wheelchair user are **import tax free and VAT free**. I did get a Can-Am quad bike imported from the USA and had a rack fitted to the back for my chair. I also had a thumb throttle and brake fitted, all of which qualified as import duty tax free and VAT free as it was then classed as a motor vehicle for a wheelchair user as it had been adapted.

Summary: So there are some perks. I know this is a fast and loose term to use given the situation but why not enjoy some of the advantages of the crappy situation? Honestly, I found it keeps me I would like to say, sane but I know my family and friends may say, was he ever? Lol!

13. THE PAPERWORK

One of the more daunting and annoying tasks, but it is paperwork and once it is out of the way, it is done.

Now they do offer help with this should you need it, I have found the forms to be ghastly worded and sometimes slightly (well, I will just say it as it is) worded awfully and f*****g painful as you are explaining the most intimate details about yourself to a complete stranger. Then if they don't understand, a follow up call which has happened in the past. However, I now fill them out like I'm explaining it to a child or in a very simple format. I do get letters from my doctor, physio and also the psychologist. This helps fill in some of them as they are 'to whom it may concern' but can help with medical terminology and wording.

Note: This is now all switching over to Universal Credit slowly but surely, but the questions have to be filled out honestly and with a harsh truth. This is why I personally found it painful as while I try to live as independently as possible, there are limits and you have to give the brutal truth.

I have used these letters myself for 3 majors forms and then some others:

DLA – now known as PIP (Personal Independence Payment)
ESA – Employment Support Allowance
Housing Benefit and Council Tax Relief – now UC (Universal Credit)

The forms are annoying to fill out and as I say, my advice would be to have someone with you – friend or family when filling them out and getting your letters in advance can be helpful. I keep a file medical/form file, so it is all in one place and ordered.

Once you have completed these forms if you need to you can also use the outcome if applicable, for other government departments and private companies, such as:

Student Loans Company
Council Tax reduction
Motability Scheme
Blue Badge Scheme

These also come in handy if you see something you wish to apply for such as a job or grant to start own business or work from home set up, etc. So keeping on top of the paperwork is key. While annoying, I do find ringing the departments beneficial to keep them on track and ask questions about the process status and my place in the queue as if you leave it, while they do get round to it, most of the above are understaffed so it does keep it on track.

Summary: OK, paperwork is always going to be a pain in the backside but the framework above – file at the ready, makes it less of a pain. Every year for the first 3–4 years you have a review. With these documents at the ready, though it cannot completely smooth out the process, it does as they say, takes out the potholes! No unforeseen bumps.

Note: This government-run benefit system is always changing, and goalposts are always moving. Hence why keeping on top of things and informed of the changes is a very good idea.

14. FINANCES

Money, money, money. Being disabled gets expensive really quickly if you're not careful.

My first piece of advice would be, if you have newly found yourself in a wheelchair and you know you are in it for the long haul by means of chair and hospital stays, is to cut away any and all unnecessary expenses you may have. I was lucky as my university reacted very quickly to the situation only knowing I had had a serious accident. They put a hold on everything. My TV provider, phone company, landlord, and my insurance company, all were informed by phone and via email about the situation that I was currently in, and things were shut down or at the very least, slowed or placed on hold. This was all with the help I believe of my mother and my partner who were staying in my flat while I was in hospital.

My second piece of advice from experience is – don't do what I did. Buying things I just didn't need or were only useful for a really short period, I nearly burnt though ten years of savings before I got to know myself again. Most of the things were not helpful in the slightest. Now you could say this is down to being naive and, being blunt to a degree yes, I fell for products, potions, pills and lotions – a complete waste for the most part. Also 'specially made' memory foam cushions are just the same as memory foam cushions but the uplift in the price tag for disabled people is quite frankly disgusting and to this day make me angry.

It is a very unregulated marketplace which makes my blood boil, and I will do something about this. (Wait and see.)

Wheels for my chair and inner tubes is another example. Wheelchair companies for the most part are fair about prices but if you look at the tyres and the inner tube, they're the same as a child's racing bike tyre. There's no difference between even the brand name! And fitting costs less for a child's bike. So you go from a bill of £150.00 for a pair of wheels from a supplier marketing to the disabled, to £45.00 plus £10.00 for fitting at a bike shop or Halfords for example. I won't name and shame these companies because of the simple fact you can now Google this information.

Bearings for your casters for the two small wheels on the front of the chair is another good example. If you're confident in popping out the old ones and pitting in the new ones. A wheelchair company charges £30.00 for a total of 4 bearings. On eBay £12.99 plus shipping for a bag of 20! And this probably takes an hour the first time you do it. The second time, half an hour. These are examples of two small aspects of the cost of wheelchairs.

In regards to management of your bills and finances, it is also a balancing act, and it is worth speaking to a accountant that can advise in these matters. There is information online but be aware that not everything you read is 100% accurate. Even some things in this book may be out of date and irrelevant by the time it is published but apply a good grounding of common sense, ask for help where required, there is no harm in that.

Summary: You know the saying, 'work smart, not hard'? This would be good regarding the point that most of the components on your chair are, unless custom-made are standard fittings and usually found in other cheaper products and also can be bought and stored. Then when the need arises… well there you go, another small thing. Read the manual for the wheelchair or Google the pdf or watch a few videos on YouTube that can save you a lot of time and money and also helping form you own list of what you may need, parts and otherwise.

15. CLOTHING

As I said, you will save money on shoes at the very least!

I will start with under layers – bit pants but yes, **pants** or **boxers** or **underwear** whatever you wear underneath. Size up. Why? Well you don't want things tight especially if they are elastic at the top. If too tight, they can cause a pressure sore or rub and cause damage. Better to have not too loose but not tight to cause red marks. You will see this in a day. If too tight, it is important to keep an eye in your skin in all areas daily.

Socks – This may sound silly but yes, socks. I used to wear just normal socks but if you have been injured like me, e.g. no use of legs, you have probably been given a lovely pair of what can only be described as stockings just coming above the knee. The good news is this is temporary. The other good news is you can take away something with this. Wearing taller, thinner socks helps with your feet swelling. I say thinner as your feet will still swell but this slows it down. And being thinner allows things not to rub then they do proactively protect your skin and ankles.

Tops – Again this is dependent on your level and condition. For me, it was a switch from button shirts to T-shirts (soft ones). This is because of the hypersensitive band I described around my chest. I still wear buttoned shirts – a size larger again but with a T-shirt underneath.

Jeans or joggers – Ha, now this this a learning curve. If you have been stuck in joggers for the whole of your hospital stay, you guessed why – it's to protect you skin, easy to take off and so on. Now assuming you wish to get back into jeans or normal trousers, there are some starting tips. Nothing with buttons on the back or on the bum area as you don't want to be sitting on them all day. Also if you do find some without buttons, get a size larger and leave the top button undone so they are not tight or rubbing, Another part is if they have back pockets, do either one of these two things. Watch your skin carefully as you should be anyway, making sure the seam is not too thick and causing damage. If not, all good but do keep an eye out for it. The other alternative it to take the back pockets off! Then there are no seams. You can go even one step further and have jeans with jogger tops but to be honest, I haven't had to travel that path. I did consider it and do think it is handy to know about.

Dressing smart, apart from a suit jacket I found most clothes however to need little to no modification and the only reason I had my suit jacket tailored was simple. One the sides would get dirty rather quickly and two, I simply got fed up with making sure it was tucked in.

Summary: Now style and fashion is a subjective field. I love nice clothes; I enjoy keeping myself looking smart, and it makes me feel good. This is just a small aspect but makes the world of difference in my opinion, as feeling smart or good just makes you feel better. It does for me, plus boy or girl who doesn't wanna look good? Don't get me wrong, some days I just wanna crash out in joggers or pjs but hey, this is just my point of view. Do what makes you feel comfortable – that is probably the main takeaway.

16. CHANGES TO LOOK OUT FOR

Mentally, physically, socially, and in your routine.

Mental changes: I have faced or have had to is being frustrated about simple things. My patience levels shot down. I have always been the type to want things done like it was yesterday. But this is part of my own make-up. Having been a chef and pushed very hard to change my career at a later stage in life, (also with my plans I would set a goal and complete it) I have had to learn, much to my annoyance that this is a double-edged sword. I have had to focus the frustration and channel it to the right path as sometimes I would notice I could catch myself taking it out at the wrong person or object. I did set myself some ground rules, but I did notice a large shift in how I had to approach things especially with people around me. Objects don't get hurt feelings which is a small blessing. With this destructive nature, I have learned to let out, like a pressure valve. I found it would build up in the background. I became aware of this, then I would learn what I should be looking out for!

 The/or a solution – Find a way to have an outlet both physically and a mentally. By this I mean taking a sledgehammer to something and smashing it up can be such a release. After doing this simple task, I write down how I was feeling and sometimes surprised myself in what I wrote. It tapped into the mental side my brain. I had time to process what I was feeling and why as I was smashing something, just focussed on the act. Guess it was one of my forms of odd meditation. (Note: Safety goggles required, lol.)

Now I apply this to new things such as clay shooting or rifle target shooting as one, when you point and bang and hit a clay and two, where you have to think about the sun the wind the distance allowing myself to be adsorbed by the moment. Another would be simple woking out or even just writing down what I felt. I know there is an odd thing to keeping a journal but hey if it works, why not.

Physical: Massive change has already happened if you have a spinal cord injury like me, it is a given. The small but most significant change can happen up to 2 years after injury. But like a newly built house, it takes time to settle into place. It doesn't mean you can't move in; it just means you may see a new crack or hear a creak in the frame or floor. To come out of the metaphor, this is when you are healing still and nerve endings – those 120 billion signals are a adjusting both at the point of injury and in your brain. It is rewiring itself to learn new patterns on a physical level, subsequently you find things change. Look out for both the good as well as the bad changes. Both are just as important for me. It was not till 8 months after my injury I noticed some of my stomach and back muscles where still working and I could with focus, trigger them to work. This helped me with my balance greatly, but it wasn't a straight line. There were parts that did and others that didn't.

A negative or I suppose a bad change was temperature control became worse. So I found that over time, with hot and cold air temperature I would take longer and longer to react to. Then also recovery from the biggest change I found was not being able to regulate my temperature between 12–16°C.

One minute I was freezing, the next I was too hot. It is still like this. I haven't pushed to try and solve it as to be honest while slightly annoying, I don't fancy medication for it or messing about with it as it can be handy in some ways.

(Good book: David Eaglman, "Livewired" explains more about the brains approach to some of the above topics.)

Changes in your social habits can be because of physical or mental impairment. I found I lost a few 'friends' and not just because I can be an ass!

Socially it comes in some waves, I think there is not a right way or wrong way of doing it but throwing yourself back into the 'normal' world can feel very different. Also you face the questions and the looks. Bearing in mind that prospect can be too daunting. Then there is the other option, of slowly moving back into normal social circles again. This is all down to personal choice and let's face it, we do live in a very strange and crazy world these days. Is there ever a 'normal' one?

One warning of social change to look out for is people introducing themselves as new friends or advisors. I treat people with fairness but over social media platforms especially some of the messages I have received are clearly scams or con artists. The same with emails and one or two people who try in person to take advantage. I have found these people work in groups targeting key words or certain comments on social media. With these people I assume a blunt position, expressing my concerns at the very start. A non-scammer wouldn't be phased by this. Some go a little quiet. Those you are face-to-face with are more experienced and will let this carry on and try bluffing, though it is shameful behaviour. But I make sure they leave with a lasting impression that I'm not to be f*****d about with should it come to light they are trying a scam. This doesn't mean all people are scammers. Some do care and offer help; hence I give them a chance and be blunt not rude, but you can be seen as a soft target when having a disability. Make sure they know you are not.

Routine: Noticing a change in routine not self-introduced but that has just happened, e.g. going to bed earlier and getting up later. It could be that you are just over doing it and need that little extra time. It is also worth noting that something like the above can also be triggered by your emotional state even if you are not aware, so it is key to address it. Note it and question why it may be. The same goes for eating. This can also be a noticeable change to look out for. I don't like the idea that sleeping more means you're automatically depressed. It just isn't that simple. It can be that you have been over doing it and need to take a day, think it through it all and if it is something deeper, it may be worth addressing with someone. Sometimes these small changes even just talked about can resolve themselves, but routine is very dependent on how you choose to live your life.

Summary: All of the above are just small things that can make a big difference in the end, and they again are my personal perspective and approach. Like any and all advice, it is subjective to your situation. I hope there are parts you can find helpful within it, even if you do not have a spinal cord injury but are a wheelchair user.

17. FINDING YOUR NEW INTERESTS AND HOBBIES OR WORKING OUT A WAY TO CARRY ON WITH OLD ONES

I was very active both physically and I suppose mentally. I enjoyed many things including motorbike track days, go-karting, off-road biking, skiing, swimming, climbing, travelling, running and I also worked. I loved to work. On a non-physical aspect, I enjoyed night photography, taking things apart and putting them back together (like my first car) then also reading, drawing, painting, designing things, cooking and generally being outdoors.

I found once bound to the wheelchair it was like, "Oh no," from the doctors and OTs, "You can't do that." I just wouldn't accept it so I found new ways to do pretty much everything on the list above (minus the running) but just either in a different way or making any adaption so I could.

Motorbiking and track days is an interesting one. There are two ways you can do this. One is my own design, which isn't publicly available yet. Or two, you can adapt your bike with a thumb throttle and brake and Kliktronic gear shifter which shifts your gears at the push of a button, then toe clips for your boots. I did used to have special boots, but I realised a small plate of steel with an ankle brace or lip and a racing bike toe clip actually worked better. I also Velcro my legs to the bike at the knees and inner thighs and to the catch and release method at the front and back of the bike and then simply do as I said. As you pull away, you're off. Coming to a slow, they catch. It does take practice but some offer this as experience days. (My system for my bike means I don't need people to help me. It isn't publicly available yet story tbc one day.)

Go karting: Few places have hand controls, but they are around. I've found a place in Milton Keynes to be the best so far. The transfer is very tricky, so it is worth practicing floor to chair transfers first.

Swimming: The oddest sensations with my disability. Weightlessness is just better than lying in bed and swimming does the world of wonders for my back! It took some practice using only my upper body. People seeing me without a shirt felt a little scary at first but that got forgotten about as soon as I'd had my first swim.

I tried the mono-wheelchair skiing. I also used to snowboard as well. It was easy and fun. Hard to remember not to flop over at the bottom and brilliant for balance however for me it felt time to turn the page. I just couldn't go as fast as I used to, however it's amazing what some people can do. But as I write this, I am reconsidering it as I have seen a mono-chair board and people using kites. That mixed together looks as if it could be fun!

Travelling: OK, so I used to travel a lot when I was younger and a young man. Even now I still do, it just involves a lot more planning and paperwork. There was an article about it some time ago in the

SIA healthcare magazine (I will talk about the SIA later on in the helpful links section). It can be done and is still every bit as fun!

Just being out and about 'walking' (well, rolling but I still call it walking though) with my dogs or while listening to some tunes either for pleasure or fitness reasons is enjoyable. Put on a free wheel and it's hard to find a spot I can't get into.

I now also go shooting more, both clay and target shooting. I used to shoot for fun every now and then, but I think I'm a member of three clubs now and love the good day out either in a group or on my own.

Working out how to make all this possible was an interesting one. I did have clear information from the spinal centre but me being me, I wanted to go further and also wanted to improve my balance and also strengthen the shoulders and wrists. Before my accident I was probably in the fittest, best condition of my life possibly about 79 kg or 12.5 stone and not an inch of fat on me. I was playing rugby and also a lot of the other physical actives I've mentioned. When I left the spinal centre I was probably just under 60 kg or 9.5 stone – that's being generous as I was so skinny. The combination of hospital food, lack of exercise and total mind f*** was all it was, plus the huge amount of medication just killed my appetite. I also had a change in some tastes. I changed from tea to coffee for some reason, but that is not the point. The weight drop wasn't acceptable to me and I knew wrists and shoulders were now going to need to be protected with a healthy layer of muscle. Remember, when you're not in a wheelchair, you don't work these muscles really ever unless you specially are doing a targeted full body work out. There are many new aches and pains you will get, but this is because you're not designed to constantly sit.

However, the good news is I targeted these areas that were hurting, e.g. being over-worked, learned how to stretch and focus on the areas that would keep my posture good and my core healthy first. As I said before, you have to take ego out of the workout at the start because you do need to be able to move the next day, and it's not like you can still have an 'arm day' and then a 'leg day' and alternate.

So, yes, ego out, lower weights, higher reps, lots of work using my own body weight and a TRX movement balance ball to help with my core. This took what felt like a lifetime to sit and balance on and paddle all the way around even now, and most importantly someone to watch over me. A personal trainer sounds expensive, but it was once a week and they made sure I was keeping a good check on my movements and that I wasn't overextending any joints or about to pull any muscles. Over six months this got better, and I got more confident in myself. I soon was able to start to up the weights and build back my form. For the most part, clear changes were evident in my lats, neck, shoulders, triceps and forearms. All of this is to protect my wrists and shoulders for as long as possible and to be able to cover the weight of my own body when required, which if you want to do floor to chair transfers frequently, it's best to train for it.

I would take Velcro straps and a weight belt to the gym. This was sometimes to balance me or just to keep my legs out of the way or if the weight I was pushing up or pulling down would be exceeding my own body weight, as you can't grip with your legs and you shoot off. I learned this the hard way. It is also a useful and funny way to know your own body weight as scales don't really exist for wheelchair users. Well they do but they are really expensive and just not for me.

So in non-physical hobbies there's not too much of a change for me; just takes little more planning though.

Cooking is all still doable. I found though if the kitchen floor isn't raised, chopping is an issue although two thick folded tea towels and the right wooden chopping board to do the job just fine. In cheffing you have to have what they call a 'shit pot'. It's the tops and ends or peelings of whatever you're preparing. It comes in handy when chopping away instead of trying to also have a bag or be near the bin, etc.

Photography: I use a tripod which was like the one I already had but lightweight, and I made a strap to carry it. Most won't fit in a backpack or will hit the wheel of the chair so I have it on my lap. To stop it flying off, I strap it to my jacket using Velcro because if you fall out of your chair, you don't want to land on the tripod – its pointy. Velcro because 9/10 it pulls apart. This also applies to things in your jacket pockets! Nothing pointy. I learned this the hard way, now hopefully you don't.

Painting: With a couple of bits of wood I fashioned the right height stand for my painting as sitting makes that a little harder, but this was my work around. The difference I found was remembering to wear an apron that covered my knees and feet and not leaving anything I could knock over with the chair on the floor.

Reading/writing/drawing (or any sitting activities): I find these best to do out of the chair either on the sofa or on the bed. The reason being posture; sitting so you're not leaning over the book, laptop or sketch pad, keeping an eye on yourself and remembering to also move (pressure relief) is important. Through practice this becomes second nature but at first I would need a timer reminding me.

Note: These are just a few of many activities you can do and try but not everyone is going to like the same thing. The main essence is doing it safely as it can be done, keeping a good eye on your skin and posture. None of the above really takes a lot of work for myself as I do not want to become hunched over or get a painful neck. The pressure relief is one that with time, comes as second nature. Working out I do as much as I can to keep my back strong and core working as best it can.

I also find some activities are good in a group and some solo. I like shooting in a group with people there not to help me or assist but to have a good laugh with and in the club I'm a member of, its a good laugh. I haven't brought it up in detail for the safety reason and also licenses have to be obtained which are not tricky to obtain but the best start is going and joining a club or going to an open day.

Summary: As I have said, many of the activities listed are not for everyone. I am still finding new ones and it is that simple – finding what you enjoy and a way to do it. Just never give up on trying. It can be annoying and hard work but being happy is so key to lowering pain levels, keeping active and so many other benefits.

18. BRAIN FOOD

Keeping your brain active when your body is not.

This is a key thing. Sometimes you need a day or longer when you're physically tired or for some other reason in bed. Keeping your brain active in this time is important.

If that is learning a new skill or language or planning something for the future, it is important. I have found that it is best to keep your brain as active as possible in these times. I have personally seen people have more a lengthy healing time because they haven't kept their brain active, and they shift or slip into a rut. It is easily done but harder to get out of.

By falling into a rut I mean allowing yourself to give up hope of getting out of the bed and back to life. It is very different for everyone and for some it can be not a fall into a pattern but a fear of the new life on wheels. There is no judgement in this, but it is important to address it as soon as you spot it and speak to someone about how you are feeling **(this would be what people mean by mental health awareness)**. It only takes a short fall into a rut or a having down spiral. I have felt this happen to myself in a way like this. I fell into a pattern rut in late spring just after my accident. I took a taxi that had a ramp taxi (I am not a fan) but I had to go to the vets, so I took it on the way back again, same taxi. The driver thought he could just let go of the chair and I would roll backwards down in a straight line, It happened in what seemed like slow motion. He let go, the chair hit the side, the ramp came off I landed on my backside coccyx. On the upside it didn't hurt but I had one hell of a headache. I was wearing very thick jeans and that was probably a good thing. After an ambulance had attended, I was deemed fit to go home. I wasn't broken. My hand was OK; a bit scraped and sore but not too bad. I got inside and found I had scuffed my coccyx and there was a good bruise forming. The skin was ever so slightly damaged – broken not bleeding but like a carpet burn. This quickly became a problem, and it was nearly a whole summer on my side and being very careful when using the loo. The dressing had to be changed daily, creams had to be applied and the district nurse had to visit weekly. The tiny, small patch got deeper before it healed, and it took ages to heal. I was skimming a pressure sore, but it was nine weeks to heal! Ahhhh, that idiot taxi driver! Laying on my side swapping sides every so often or laying on my front was annoying. At the time, I lived in a flat overlooking the sea and I was missing the sunshine. So not fun and all because of an idiot taxi driver.

One – I don't ever take cabs with ramps anymore.

Two – I tell you this because it shows just how easy it is to damage an area of skin.

Three – This time spent on my sofa was painstakingly annoying and watching daytime TV or old movies quickly started to make me feel down.

But I started to feel I needed a task or something to do, so I found something. If I hadn't, I would have gone nuts or ended up depressed about my situation. I decided to find three tasks I could do through the day – read, draw and also take clocks apart and put them back together. They were old brass ones I brought off eBay. Staying inside and keeping all pressure off my coccyx was so tricky but it was the first time I noticed how easy it would be to just switch off and give up. I was lucky as I spoke about my annoyance and frustration at my situation to the nurse and took her advice which was the above. Start small.

Getting into a rut – well, not for me. While I did feel like this at some points, as I say I kept busy, and I think that is why I kept my brain active. I also listed the things I would do once healed and free to get back into the chair and back to the gym for longer than 10–15 minutes! But this whole summer was an eye-opener for me. My back hurt more, my head always hurt, and my mood was certainly not the best, but you have to push on and get through these things.

Summary: Keeping your brain active can keep you active later. Sounds simple but it's quick to burn through old movies or TV shows but keeping your brain fed for lack of a better term, can be more important than anything.

Note: I never had this in the spinal centre as I was careful with my skin, and I kept busy trying to break out (lol) and learn as much as possible as quickly as possible. This just gave me an insight in to how mentally easy it is to find that rut and how hard it can be to drag yourself out. But no harm in being told by the nurses that came out. They were lovely and suggested things for me new to try or read and I kept my brain healthy and fed.

19. SEX. YES!

- Openness with your partner.
- Back to school – explore your mind and body.
- Things that have changed.
- Be OK with trial and error.

OK, awkward subject? Did you just shift in your chair? I did, partly because I know my mother and father will undoubtedly read this along with my friends but it's only natural, so why not talk about sex?

Sex is such a loaded word and thought when you have been placed on two wheels or have a disability of any kind. Even broaching the subject makes some blush, but it's a function of how babies are made or for just the fun of it and it can still be very fun!

I speak as someone who was 24/25 when I had my accident which landed me on wheels and I'm now 36. I am male but I want to try and keep this chapter as gender neutral as possible – female or male or other (so many different terms now), trying to keep it as clear as possible.

Firstly, never blush at asking about it to any medical professional as they have seen and heard it probably all before or watched 50 shades of grey, ha-ha! Mind you, we shall not go into whether you have a fully kitted out red room and love grey ties, male or female… cough! (This comment is specially for the one person who gave me good non-NHS advice on the matter).

Openness with your partner is just common sense for both involved. While some find it hard to talk about and be honest, it is very much like being naked and exposed. There is absolutely no reason to feel any shame or embarrassment. Just explain how you feel or are feeling beforehand and in the moment and where you are on your new path. In fact, I have found discussing the issues with my partner to the point of where I take the worst component out of the situation which is stress or worry.

These two things before leading into sex or sexual activity of any kind will probably kill it and the mood so having an open and frank talk about where you are and how you are feeling sounds wishy-washy and soft, but it isn't. It is being prepared and also working out how to both enjoy the experience as much as possible, baby making or not. No harm in that.

Back to school with your body – I think this sentence makes it clear. Your body may have changed, your sensations or tastes may have but knowing this, is releasing. What areas feel good, and which feel bad are important; it is like creating a new road map. How many people wish they had one! This is a good reason to make one so take advantage of this situation and make your road map to feeling good. Knowing what will or won't feel good will help with being open about likes and dislikes.

Things that have changed – There may be different or new things and that is normal. Changes happen over the course of your lifetime anyway and tastes change. This is again a change that you are dealing with because you have to. But you don't. You are still in control of the situation and how you best wish to deal with it.

Being OK with trial and error – Mistakes or miss calculations can happen and knowing you're in a safe space so if things do go wrong as they do, it's not the end of the world. This happens to everyone regardless of ability/disability. I would say being prepared for it can't hurt and the mind boggles at how many people would like the benefit of hindsight or a do-over (no pun intended), Well, this is your first time again in a way,

The part to understand is male or female, sex isn't just about your downstairs parts, it's your whole body and mind. While this sounds 'hippy-ish' and probably strange, it is why it is best to talk about it all with your partner first. Last thing you want to be is uninformed and unprepared, making what should be a fun time into a stressful one.

Speaking personally on the subject of sex, it is all a matter of personal preference, knowing before you try and taking it slow. Also you don't just have to jump in there and be too hasty – as soft as this sounds coming from a 36-year-old male. Find a position just to lay. A kiss and a cuddle is a good starting point which sounds easy but finding a comfortable position just for this simple act of embrace with your partner can be difficult but not impossible.

Notes:

- Feel your skin/body total body – Where is good, where is bad.
- Work out the movement you have and what positions you are most comfortable in.
- Setting: Before you start either talking about it or even doing it, your surroundings are important, whether you're going to have your chat or have a trail setting.
- Being open: Talking about what is possible and what isn't yet on the cards, e.g. what you are willing to both try. It takes two to tango.
- Talking about sex with a sexual psychologist: This can be a good move for both you and your partner. Do your research

into it – and I don't mean porn! It may be a stimulant but not an educational tool.

Understanding changes and accepting them or allowing yourself too is one thing, but also giving your partner time to adapt is just as important. The key word here is patience. The saying, 'good things come to those who wait' crosses my mind but not always. While this can be true, understanding of the fact that you or your partner may not want to wait so, talk about it.

Summary: Anyway it unfolds or goes, don't worry there is always another day and a different way to try. Like most things and without being crude about it, it still can be as fun if not more so as you open yourself up on a whole new level that you never would have thought of before.

Last thought – Baby-making. This is all very dependent on your situation. It may still be possible, or it may not be in the traditional sense. You must be checked out and know where you are. The other part is protection. Do still use it, not only if you just don't want children but also STIs. That doesn't change regardless of your ability to be able to make a baby.

20. SHARING

Lighter topic. Less thought required. Things I have messed up on and what I learnt from that. Basically, I have cocked up and what I have learnt, so a point of view of what not to do.

Velcro to shoes on foot plate — So, my feet would fall off and I could drag one in front or worse under the chair which is not good. I thought Velcro to the base of my shoes and on my foot plate would work. It did but then as I was getting out the chair, my shoes would stay stuck on it. Yeah, didn't work.. funny. But a slight adjustment to the angle of the foot plate and calf strap was all that was needed.

Not checking brakes on the chair — Forgetting that the chair can fly away from you, and you end up on the floor. So check the brakes.

Thinking that it will be OK without preparing first — Don't go out without the disabled badge or backpack. Better to keep that on you. Also having an empty spare 2 litre bottle in the car can come handy if it's a long drive.

When using a disabled loo, make sure the door is locked, also that someone hasn't wrapped the red cord emergency on the bar next to the loo. You don't want that being pulled.

Not calling first, going to a new place or area and having either a look on Google street view or booking a hotel through a website. I have turned up at places and not been able to get into a room. This could have been simply averted with a phone call or email to the place to check it all out first.

Labradors – Using them like husky's to pull you along with a body harnesses. Mine are not trained to do this but I'm sure they could be but if both your hands are on leads, you can't stop!

Stopping quickly – OK, if you are going to go out for a big push, while not stylish, wear gloves, especially if it is cold. But if you want to come to a sudden stop, the extra grip from gloves can come in very handy and also not give you a friction burn which really hurts like a paper cut.

Making sure your car is off before getting in – Don't blow up your engine! The car has to be off as you enter legs in first with an easy transfer. What can happen is your foot slides on to the accelerator pedal which is not the best. The car could be off down the road, or you could be revving the engines nuts and bolts off. Taking your time to transfer is another good point. There is no point rushing it.

Night lights – The amount of times I have been tripped up by a dog toy or shoe or box in the night. I am a bit of a night owl and instead of using the insanely bright light on my phone or something else, a dim nightlight is well worthwhile getting.

Forgetting your phone – just don't.

Sitting on something you have put on top of your chair like keys, phone, pencil/ pens, book – Sounds stupid but you don't want the thing imprinted on your legs or ass for a week afterwards or worry about getting a pressure sore from it same goes for in bed.

Dinner tray or protection for legs with hot things. Place nothing hot on your lap from a cup of coffee to a dinner plate! As I explained earlier in the book, this can burn you and you won't know it. In regards to coffee or tea, ask for two large paper cups and fill halfway not to the brim. The double layer stops you getting burnt also gets you from A to B half full means you don't spill anything.

The double-check before bed sounds again stupid but it is an odd situation granted but going for the loo just before bed and not forgetting can make a world of difference. And remembering to cut down drinking early in the evening 2 hours before bed that or set an alarm.

Allowing extra time to get in and out the car if you're going somewhere. Practice getting your chair in and out the car smoothly stops you from rushing and bashing it into everything. I personally allow an extra ten minutes either side of a trip for the chair if I'm by myself.

Falling for disabled friendly products. So these are many and at a premium cost. Nine times out of ten I found they don't do as they say and cost a fortune compared to something that is exactly the same but not aimed at disabled people.

Forgetting to look at the ground for bumps, curbs and stones. This will depend on your casters – the two smaller front wheels. If they hit a bump or stone and you're not ready, it can send you flying so keep an eye out.

Rolling backwards – I have managed to roll back and subsequently came off a curb or into someone not prepared. `Looking over your shoulder isn't a bad idea.

Remember every action has an equal and opposite reaction. Vacuuming or sweeping can be done but when on wheels if you push one way with a broom or vacuum cleaner, you're going the other way! The solution is simple – turn sideways. I tried pulling the cleaner along and strapping it to the front. All I ended up with was a scratched skirting board or an unswept or cleaned carpet.

Mud! OK, if it is wet and you're going to go through puddles or mud there's two options: Have some wipes by the door and a bin bag or put in the wheel guard. It will keep your trousers tidy and elbows too. You often find you will use different parts of body to stop and go. Slow the chair down if the wheels are wet or muddy and be prepared to change after, also wipes or towel can be handy.

Summary: All of the above I have messed up so these would be the hints of things to do in order to not to make the same silly mistakes I have. I am still learning and by no means will I ever stop. Just have to find new ways of doing things.

21. SOCIAL AND WORK SITUATIONS

Both social and work situations can be stressful. Remember that taking this into account before you set off has an impact not only mentally but physically. You find your energy levels change and subsequently your drinking needs change and your eating pattern changes. The changes can be slow or fast depending on the situation but knowing this is half the battle. Understanding that your energy levels are impacted by them is good. If you have kept track of things, you can be fairly certain of the impact these two situations will have on you.

For me, stress will make me need the loo more and also can trigger spasms in my stomach area, but I know this now because I have found out the hard way. It is something I now prepare for and look out for.

In overwhelming situations both at work or socially I tend to find taking 2–3 minutes very useful in not allowing panic or stress to seed itself to deep. This doesn't have to be done dramatically or rushed but knowing you can pull yourself out of a situation is important; also taking the time for yourself.

Work situations – It is best to talk to your boss and let them know they can put you in a high-pressure environment. This is different to stress. But do explain the difference and just explaining the basics openly will give you the confidence to be able to push harder and interact and learn in new ways because you have prepared for a stressful moment. When it does happen, you have the back-up if you need it or can face it and overcome it.

Social – So if it's a village green party or family or friend's birthday or a drink down the pub or a coffee with a friend or by yourself, the key is knowing what could happen. For example, the stupid questions. It is just preparing yourself and remembering to relax. Yes, the odd comment can stray your way from a complete stranger but just remember, it is your choice how you react, if at all.

Summary: This is quick and fast advice but nonetheless true. The main point is knowing how these can affect you and being prepared if it is tested. This way you limit the annoying part.

22. MOVEMENT AND EXERCISE

I did say I would back up on to this area as it is a vast area to cover, so i will try not to bore you and keep it simple or try to at the very least.

Movement: So every movement you make is going to take a toll on your joints; your back and shoulders, upper spine, neck, and wrists. It is important you practice these movements. There is a reason for this as it is to enable you to do them smoothly and with maximum efficiency. This helps protect your joints the big ones and the small ones as well. This will allow you to also protect your muscles so think of this as the everyday warm up or passive exercise for when you're just generally moving.

Exercise: This is where you actively decide to target the areas proactively to avoid injury. But with stressing the area, the important part to remember here are two areas which I would say are maintenance and conditioning.

Conditioning the muscles around your joints to protect them and making your movements. The easiest possible things you must understand are that you are building yourself up, strengthening the areas that are key to you and keeping yourself as fit as possible. This is setting the path for you to be able to capitalise on the working muscles you have left meaning your movements have strength behind them.

This is stressing the areas you need every day and you will be sore. The trick is not to be too sore that you can't move the next day. I speak from personal experience when I say it's easily over done! When you try upping the weights and stressing the muscles, as the adrenaline is pumping it's easy to get lost in the moment. Hydration is more important if you are doing this for both during and after. It will help you be less sore the next day. Also when washing, cooling the shower down is better I have found but this is personal preference. **The knock-on effects** – I have had bruising to my kidneys, pulled a lower ligament giving me a headache trying to work out how, and yes, I was barely able to move the next day.

Now the only way you are going to find this out is by pushing it but you should do it under supervision and guidance. You will soon learn you limits and then where and how far you can push beyond them. The reason for it? As I say, I was very fit before my accident and would always be a slim build but muscular. Part of it was self-image when I was in the chair but for me the main objective was to know that if I needed to have enough raw power in the tank to drag, pull myself up should I come out the chair and also have the stamina to do so. Now I can put all my body weight through one arm and wrist without worry of damage. I don't make a habit of it, but it is nice to know I have it in the tank should it be needed.

A story of why and an example of this – It would have been a few weeks ago, I went in the evening to check out some woodland I was thinking of buying. I took my normal chair and free-wheel. I drove up but it had been raining the day before and the track was a bit muddy. Not an issue as I was in the right gear – full waterproofs and I had my freewheel and backpack so I parked the car, jumped out, set up and all good. I went uphill for 30–40 metres into this wood and it started raining but it was still not a big deal. The wood was lovely, and I liked hearing the sound of rain on the trees. I was warm and not fussed if stuff in my backpack got a bit wet. Anyway, I had my peaceful moment and started going back down. Then a grass/mud track and I heard a hissing sound; nuts! My freewheel was now leaking air ok so I tried to speed up. The ground had got a bit muddier and the freewheel was now flat and my very skinny tyres started shining in the mud. The rain had now also got heavy, and I was 10–15 metres from my car. I got stuck.

Now in these moments in life sometimes you just have to say, "Oh shit." I am deep in the woods, it's also getting darker I try for a few minutes to pull back, rock forward, anything to move forward but nope, it wasn't going to happen. The chances of being found? Yes, I would be but that's going to take ages, so I put my phone away as I was going to call for help. The grass, now a mud track was mostly downhill so, being in full waterproofs, I transfer to the ground (checking for rocks) and I get my backpack on my back. I drag the chair sideways out the mud. Blimey, I had sunk. The problem was there was now no way I could get back into the chair without it just sinking in again. So I push it down the slope about 10 metres till I get to a rocky part which is better. That whole ten meters took me about 45 minutes. Me lifting my body weight slowly in the mud out and over and down. I get the chair onto the rocks/gravel, sit in and I can move over the area to the last 5 metres. I open the car door. It is now pretty dim, and I was covered in mud. I go round to the boot of the car where I have a towel and a bottle with a bit of water. I rub the wheels down and try to remove as much mud as possible. I get into the car and turn up the heating. I was covered in mud still… ha!

I had the energy and strength to do it, had a big drink of water while driving home and when I did get home half an hour later, my partner was like, "What on earth happened to you?!" I was grinning while saying it was just a bit muddy. I did explain later on what had happened and there were a few eye rolls and so on but the main thing is, I was able to get myself out because I had conditioned my body to do this.

(I know this is an extremely stupid situation to get into but I dont like asking for help; I would rather get a little muddy and also be fit enough to sort out my own stupid mess rather than call for help. But this is after years of training and also knowing I was in the right gear and if I did get really stuck, I would have called for help, regardless of my blushes!)

Maintenance exercise: This is where I do a high reps low weight or resistant bands and cardio. I do this on the muscle groups less used every day which keeps my posture good and helps relieve pain. Keeping up good cardio is important while low impact on muscles, it gets the blood pumping and keeps the heart healthy. I also swim on these days, and it allows me to stretch out and is also another form of cardio. It also highlights any core issues so if I can't balance as well, I know which areas to target and work gently on. As the muscles will be smaller and weaker, it is important to start slow on them and work them out if you have a spinal injury. If not, that won't be an issue but the principal of taking it slow, stands.

In essence, take your ego out and take it slow. It will feel so slow at first and frustrating but stick with it and don't overdo it causing damage.

Work out movements in the back e.g. starting with basics, always worth meeting a personal trainer so you get it right.

23. TRAVELLING

Travel is open to you, as I mentioned before. The difference is the list in preparation and understanding the things you may need although some things you can't plan for, so you get insurance and check the fine print (making sure you're covered with your disability). Research, as I said is all well and good – looking up hotels online and booking, but if you notice at the bottom of most websites it says and I quote, "While every endeavour is made to have a disabled friendly room, it is not guaranteed." My advice is to find the hotel you're looking at booking but then ring the hotel directly. This applies to places you may wish to visit for a day. Ask the basics – is it fully wheelchair accessible? Do you have a disabled loo? Are there steps into the building? Sounds a bit of an overkill but this can save you having an issue or feeling embarrassed when you're there. If you are in a metropolitan city area, this may be less of an issue as most cafes or restaurants do have a disabled loo, but you don't really want to be going back and forth if you can help it. Alternatively, you can plan this into your trip or a visit to a place knowing you will need to do this to access the loo.

Calls to make – doctor, for medical supplies also copy of script if taking medication across borders. A check-up doesn't hurt either should you be concerned about anything.

With regard to hotels or places – checking the things mentioned above (loos, ramps, access) and also the price. The career price is normally free or discounted.

Insurance company – whichever travel insurance company you use even if it is included in your home insurance policy, give them a bell to check if the wheelchair is covered. On the medical insurance side, it's worth checking coverage in regards to your disability.

Travel prep – the big tick off list I have. Bear in mind I am a pack rat.

Basic Travel List

Wheelchair spares

- Inner tubes × 4.
- Small tin of grease.
- 2 types of allen keys.
- Swiss army knife with screwdriver head and pliers.

Wheelchair user supplies

- Catheters – as many as you need plus 2 extra days' worth.
- Gloves if required.
- Opti-lube if required.
- Wipes.
- Black disposable bags.
- Empty 1.5lt bottle.
- Prescription of – meds plus extra.
- One medical kit for bumps scratches bruises cuts.

Basics
- If taking car power pack, tyre pump, high vis, duct tape and wd40.
- Suitcase with clothes.
- Hand back with spare set.
- Travel tech e.g. plugs and wires.

Documents
- One from doctor – medically explaining condition / copy.
- Passport plus copy.
- Driving license plus copy.
- Insurance travel and car plus copy.
- Contacts of people, hotels, numbers and emails plus copy.

The copies of each document are to be kept in a different place so if you lose a file you have a spare.

Also, a spare car key is always worth taking.

As you can see, this list is rather long, but I would rather go away knowing I have all the things I need just in case. Most of the time I haven't needed to worry about anything, and it is simple but when I have, I have been thankful I have had things with me.

Medical supplies – I have said you can take them with you, however if you don't have the car space, you can have them shipped to the hotel in advance. This service is provided by a few people. I will be honest; I always just take what I need but I have had things shipped out to me that I had forgotten. It happens.

In regards to flying and shipping your wheelchair, ensure your chair has hard tyres on, i.e. non-inflatables. My advice is to take off the brake attachments and put them in your luggage.

This means the brakes can go in the main luggage or hand luggage. This mitigates the risk of damage to the chair. In regards to the chair, sometimes you may be able to ring the airline and ask for it to be stored in the cabin which is very much at the pilot's discretion due to safety. Should the answer be a no, then it goes into the hold. It's also worth having Allen keys required to take off the brakes.

Summary: Be prepared to adapt to change and also make the calls to ensure you holiday is just that, a holiday as stress free as possible. The list, planning and calls can be a pain but better that is at home than midway through your holiday.

24. THINGS THAT JUST MAKE LIFE A LITTLE EASIER

Earbuds — Connect to your phone and allow you to be hands free. I wear mine most of the time as I hate missing a phone call. In regards to the phone settings, adjusting it so it rings a little longer is a good idea.

Notepad or diary and pen to keep handy — I also keep a copy of my prescription in the back and a document outlining my condition on the first page so if I had an accident, it would be the first thing they would find. You can also set this on your phone on medical ID.

Small medical kit in the boot of car along with a towel, a change of clothes, an empty 2 litre bottle and a full bottle of water.

Keep grabbers in most rooms at home. They're inexpensive and really hand to have about.

Setting an alarm on your phone, PC or watch as a reminder for drinking, peeing, etc. After a while you will need this less and less as it all becomes second nature.

Water bottle that can clip to the chair or hang from the back It's handy to have one that has the time and amount on it which helps you keep track.

Summary: You will hopefully expand or take out on this list to make it your own. Sometimes the little things help though, and this is a starting point.

25. PSYCHOLOGY OF YOUR OWN MAKING

Throughout this book and over the weeks I have taken to write it, I have presented you with my own personal opinions/views and perspectives. When you take this all into account, you may not see things the same way or agree with them. **By all means, the above is what you should be making. Below is mine. What's yours?**

You will have to sort through what you find helpful and what you don't. My personal psychology or philosophical view is simple, but I believe it to be true throughout every strand of my life. Whatever the problem or situation, disability or not, get as much information as possible from sources that are proven. Where you can, base your decision on that and don't look back but do remember, that you made the decision based on the information you had at the time and so never stop learning.

With people, be as open as possible without giving all of yourself away, e.g. keep lines drawn and concrete them. Stick to the areas you want to keep private; this helps me draw up a template for how to deal with people in different social settings, for example, in public, at work, in social and family circumstances. This helps me have a plan or structure enabling me to have some control over the flow of topic or conversation and if the conversation goes off, I have my lines and know how I will deal with it. If something tries to cross that line, I then have a plan.

Emotion – I am aware I probably shut myself down to a degree, but I keep a diary of how I am feeling physically and mentally, more like a log for reference and a useful tool. I also keep in my normal diary a goal at the start of each week to keep myself in the right flow or direction.

Keeping it simple with problems – I follow a system, but this is based on years of trial and error. Even before my accident and landing myself on wheels, I learnt and practiced until perfect. The same applies with problem solving. Take apart try to fix it, have a break, try to fix it and then if unable to, ask for help. As I've tried my best, I can do this head held high.

Watching my six – So, watching my back, looking out for myself both physically and mentally, taking note of what my body needs, and tasks – are they too ambitious or taxing? And mentally giving thought as to interactions I have had but not letting them get me down if they were negative. Don't get me wrong, some things are just fucking depressing but why should they drag me down? I don't let them; I move on and don't grumble.

Moaning – Don't moan. Well do, but have a good rant to yourself. Vent yes, break something… but don't go moaning about things you can't change. Not all people but some quickly get bored of this if you keep moaning about things and they view/treat you differently. A good moan every once in a while is good to either see someone professionally or away from your friends and family and talk it through before you moan. It may be something that does need dealing with but if it's in the past, keep it in the rear view and never look back. You can't change it so why moan about it? Own it – don't let it own you.

Lastly, never give up, never give in, never stop trying. You can't be beaten. If you want to know how I think, I take things as a challenge. I work the problem or the situation to my benefit otherwise what am I doing? Sometimes I will write something or someone off. That isn't giving up but rather it's cutting your losses. A tactical move which is very different from giving up. It is quitting something for a good reason. This can be painful to do but sometimes it's for the best.

Summary: So this would be my ethos, how I think psychologically and view things from my perspective in a nutshell. This isn't everyone's take on life and won't work for everyone. My advice is to steal the bits you like, learn from the bits you don't, and make your own.

26. BREAKTHROUGH TREATMENTS, NEWS AND GOOGLE

"A sausage dog walks again after having its spine regrown using stem cell treatment."

"Polish stab victim is able to feel his legs and walk and move again after having spinal cord severed."

"Treatment for people suffering with disabilities may have brain impact to treat chronic pain and maybe help with movement again"

"Paralysed people have new hope after new treatment is discovered – a gel that slows healing process of spinal cord."

These types of headline are a frequent event and over 10 years old. Don't get me wrong, the research is going on and they are discovering new methods and doing some clinical trials. However, main stem cell treatment – I am sorry to say no, I haven't seen it change yet.

No doubt it will change, and big advances have been made but these trials and headlines are not helpful on a day to day basis. Trust me, it currently is cheaper to keep you in the chair than out and we are a small market. So, less funding goes into this area of study compared to billions of funding that goes into being able to cure the common cold treating millions. Big difference in market value.

I must have had ten texts when that dog walk story headlined. I proceeded to reply, "Yes, it won't be applicable to me or anyone else for 10 years at least." I am broken from T6-L1 and that's a lot of spine to regrow or repair.

Watch out for Google articles too or clinics offering stem cell treatment abroad. I knew two people personally that have gone for it. One didn't come back, and the other lost a bucket load of money and is now broke. The impact it had was awful. Sadly, there are lots of people and companies that pray on the vulnerable especially when it comes to disability of any kind which is so wrong. But it happens every day from pills, potions, creams, treatments and healing crystals.

The same is applied to products for the disabled as half the time it is a product rebranded as a disabled aid with a healthy mark up of 300 percent. By healthy, I mean greedy. I won't tar all products that are aimed at disabled people with the same brush. Some have been genuinely developed specifically for disabled people and that is the whole reason they then cost more as the market is surprisingly smaller, but these are few and far between. I would say just keep your eyes and ears open but when it comes to parting with cash. Be careful and talk about it with family and friends. Check out its origin and product history or treatment articles.

You soon see a pattern and will be able to make an informed decision before choosing your path and your purchase proceeds. This is not only to protect yourself but also to inform people around you not to come to you with the garbage, e.g. not getting ten texts about a treatment that is still only being tested or animals or in reports that say a case study is underway.

27. HELPFUL LINKS

So mine is a spinal injury as you are aware, but here are some helpful links to companies that deal in some way with wheelchair-based clients. I recommend them as I've found them to be helpful. **Just to be clear, none of these companies have paid me to endorse them or their services/products.**

Should you be in a chair or find yourself in one and it's not your fault, knowing good legal representation is key. It is a lengthy process, but it is important to have a good recommendation.

New Law Solicitors

Helmont House, 10 Churchill Way, Cardiff CF10 2HE

Phone: 0333 003 1909

Website: https://www.new-law.co.uk

I can't recommend New Law highly enough as they take an honest, straightforward approach, in my experience. I have met a lot of solicitors, but this firm is different in the way they handle things from personal injury to medical negligence to accidents. Again, please note – this is not a paid endorsement.

If medical supplies is an issue, I have found SIA Healthcare most proficient. I spoke about this company earlier in the book.

SIA Healthcare
Website: https://www.spinal.co.uk/get-support/sia-healthcare/
Phone: 08009800501

There is also:

Aspire Healthcare
Website: https://aspirehealthcare.co.uk/contact/
Phone: 01912790989

If you are looking for someone to talk to, it is important you look out for these qualifications in a counsellor:

BSc Hons, BA, Adv Dip Couns
(BACP, Centra Accr Course)
Dip CBT(OC) Dip .APP.SS
Dip HSW
UKRCP Registered
Independent
Counsellor/Psychotherapist
BACP Accredited Counsellor

This is not a comprehensive list. Do consult a doctor beforehand as well.

Another helpful source at your disposal is online but not all of it will be helpful. Groups on Facebook with your condition can lead to helpful links, however my word of advice would be to set up a separate profile for this and take it all under caution when reading. The reason I say this is it keeps you separated from dwelling on it and also there is lot of spam and crap you don't want to be thinking about every day. Good to check-in though and then be able to check-out. This is a personal view and the approach I have taken.

Scope is another group that is worth a look:
Website https://www.scope.org.uk

For wheelchair supplies, I personally use:
https://www.invictusactive.com/about-us/

They also have some other brilliant links and advice on their website which you can explore. I have found this to be the only company offering real world advice along with brilliant customer service and support in whatever you are trying to achieve.

28. THE DIAGRAMS OF MOVEMENT

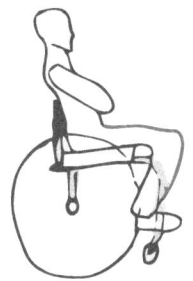 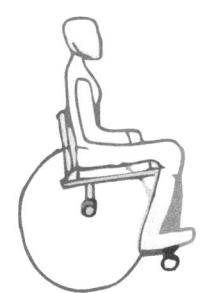

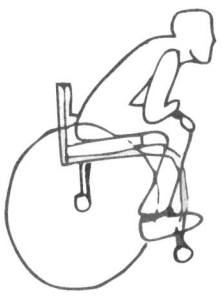 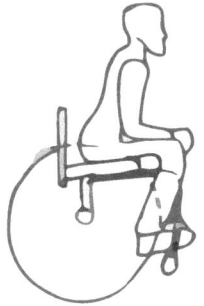

Tricks of pressure relief, the movements don't have to be drastic, it's just important you remember to do them to keep your skin in good shape and in my opinion eases pain or muscle tiredness.

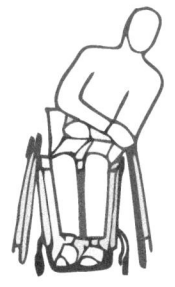 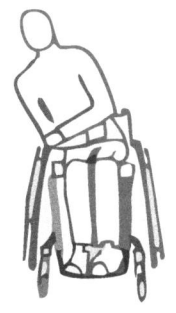

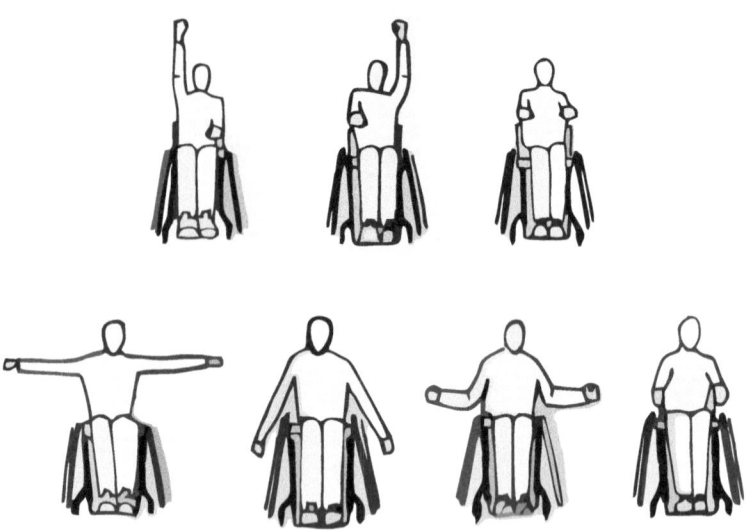

Some basic shoulder saving exercises. These protect your rotator cuffs and increase the muscle. It is best to practice with your own weight at first, then bands, and then when ready, free weights. Again, lots of reps at a lower weight, this is important as it builds strength. While I know I will say this a lot, do consult a professional.

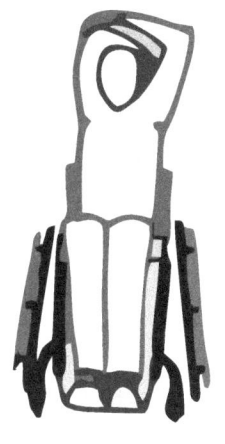
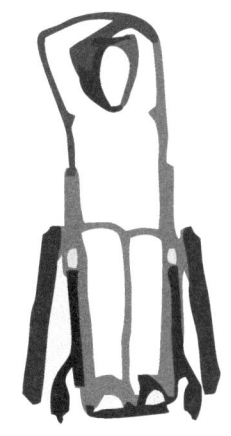
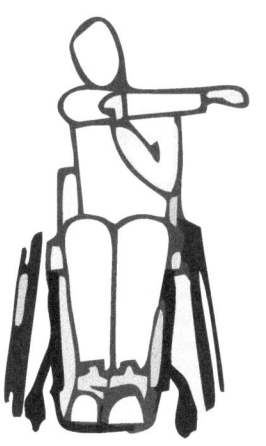

Basic stretches you can do for shoulders, triceps, and neck and back.

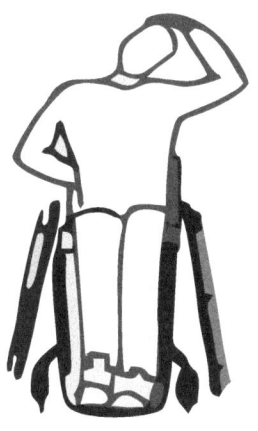

28. **THE DIAGRAMS OF MOVEMENT**

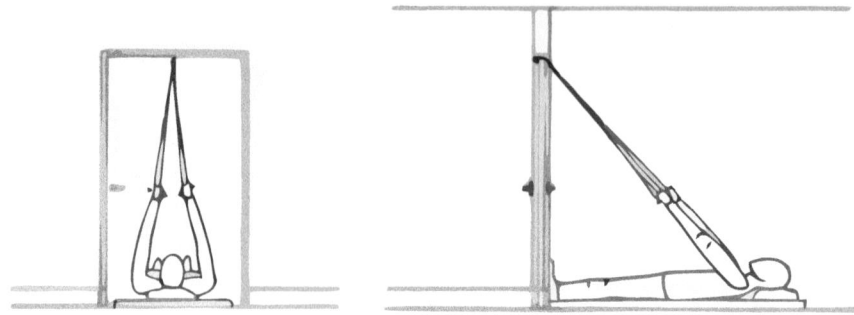

Basic TRX movements to keep good core and back strength, note the use of a mat and pillow, this helps keep your posture good, but best to be shown to a personal trainer.

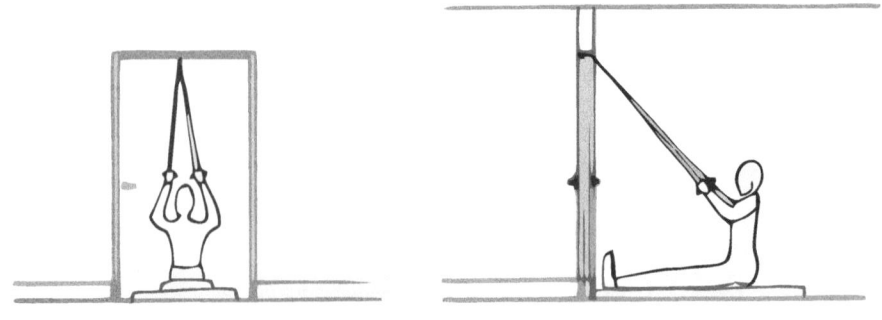

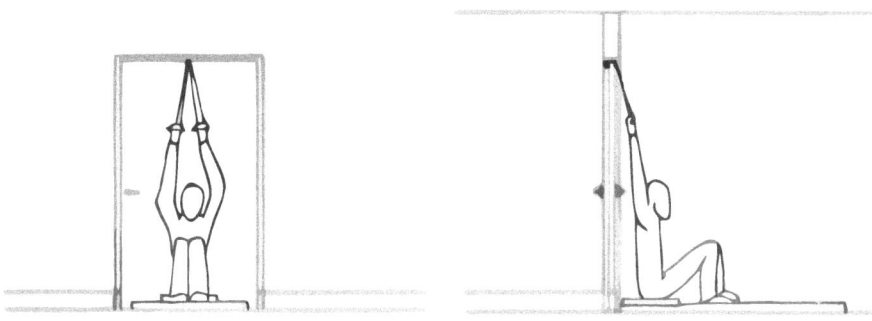

This is the more extreme TRX lift to help with shoulders. It means you lift your own body weight, the imbalance of the TRX helps, but again do consult a personal trainer. Also, the door must be smooth.

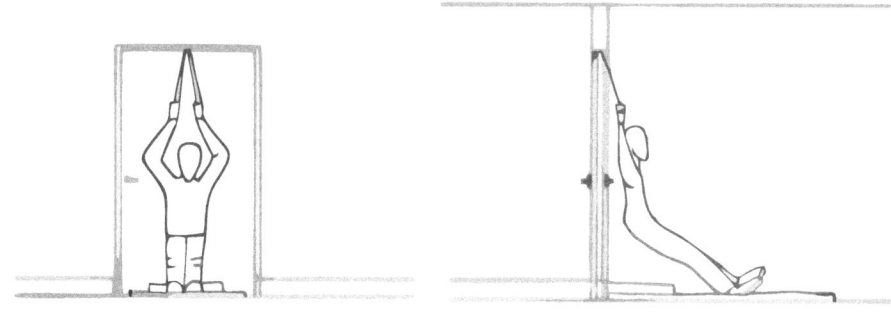

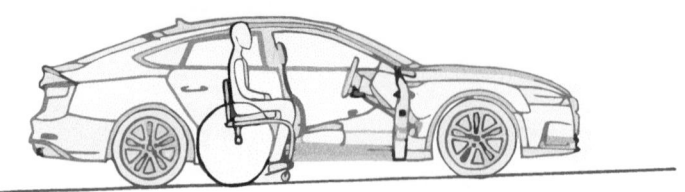

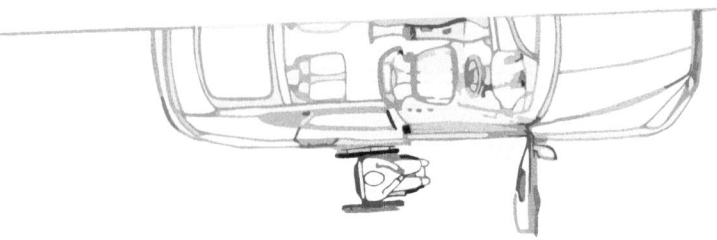

Above: Stage one is opening the car door and getting ready. This is not using a sliding board and it takes practice.

Below: Position the chair as close to the car as possible, then get legs in slow and steady with the engine off.

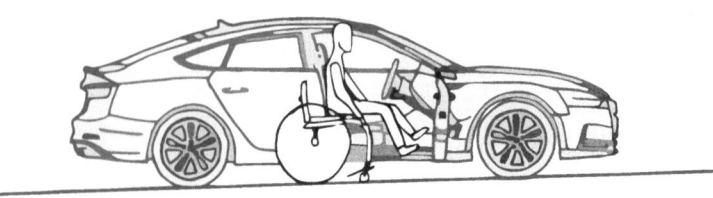

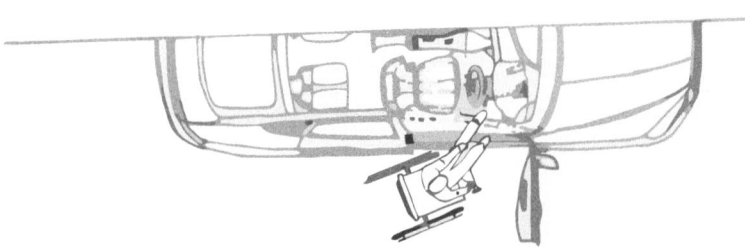

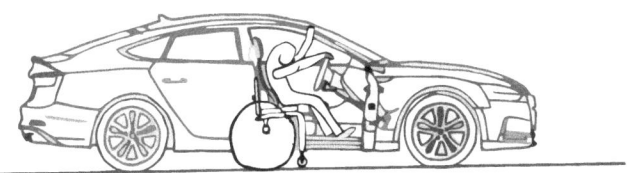

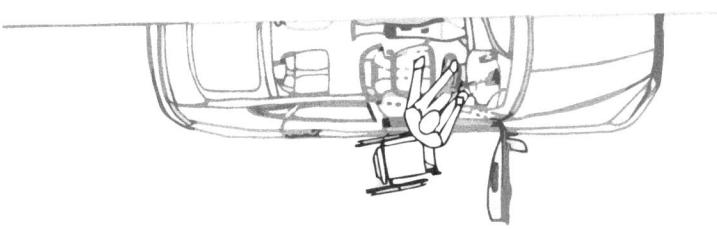

Above: Having got both legs in and half your weight, hold on to the roof handle or roof with other hand on the seat or steering wheel. Again, this takes practice and it can be done in the way you find plays to your strengths.

Below: When you're in with legs in position, now the engine can go on. It gets easier with time also getting your chair in.

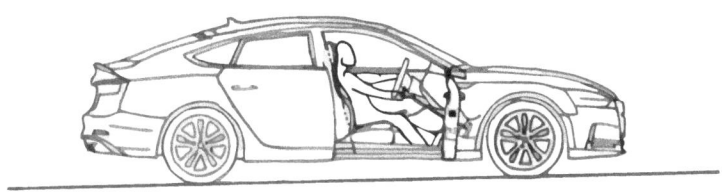

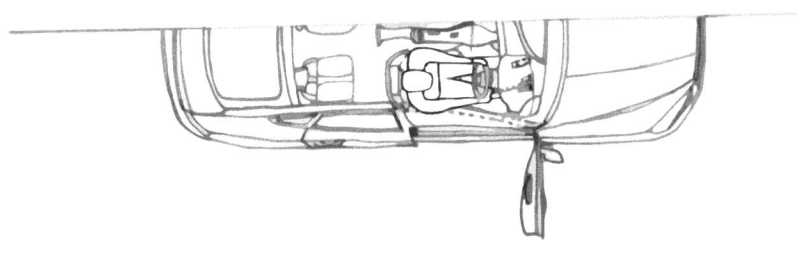

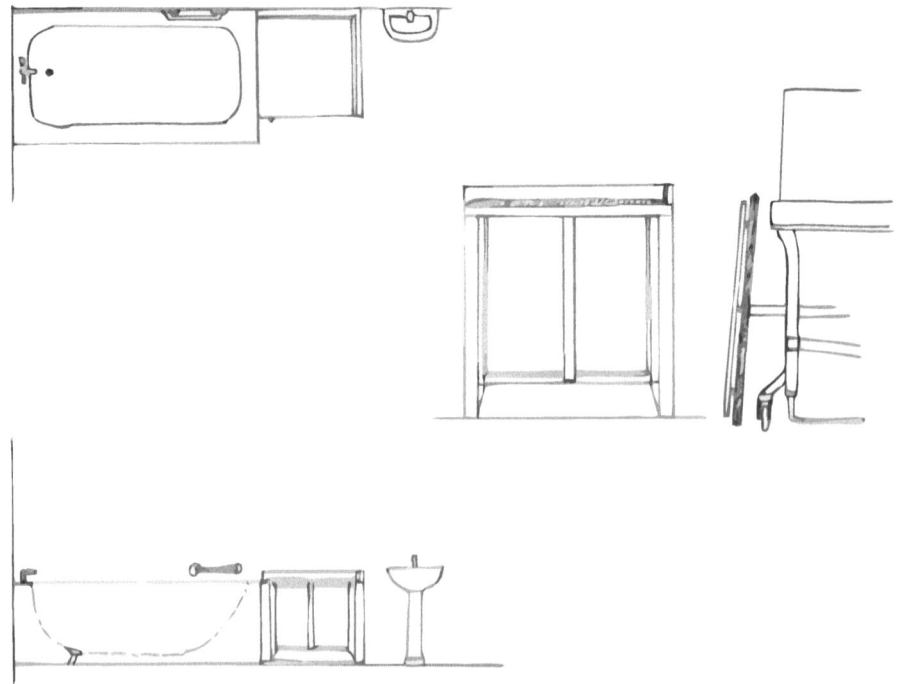

This is a plinth I made for my bathroom which also doubles up as a storage area and a way to get into the bath without a bath board due to it being the same height as the chair, and padded with a lip to stop and hold on to, it was well worth the effort.

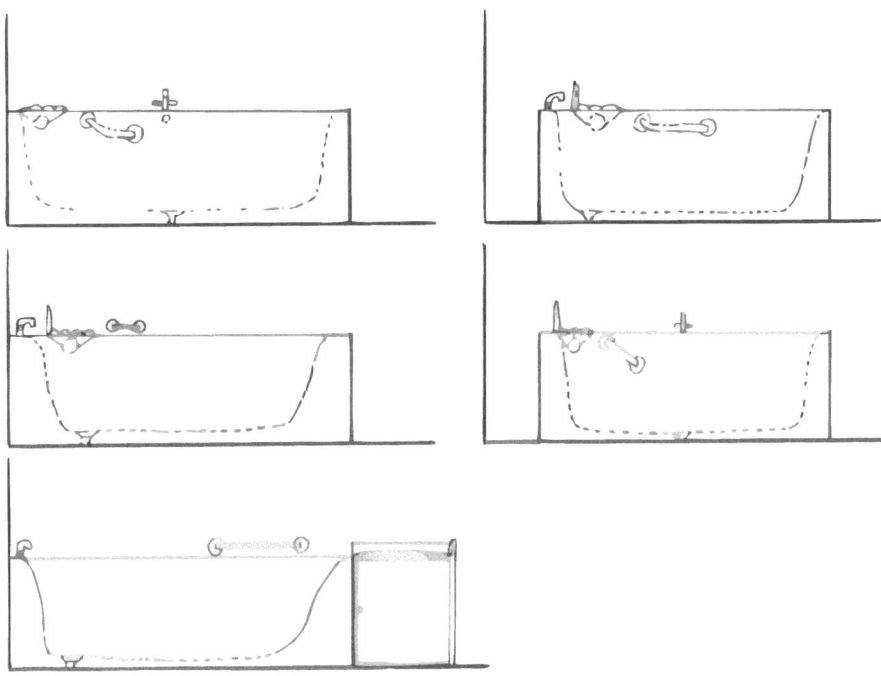

A different set up and placement of bath boards. It's best to have one with a back if near the taps. Also, best to position it as near to the wall as possible so that should you fall back, you dont hit your head.

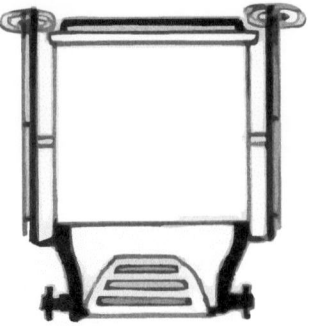

When getting out of the chair with no wall present, a simple way to get back in is to use your shoes as stoppers otherwise when transferring from the floor to the chair it can move, even with breaks on!

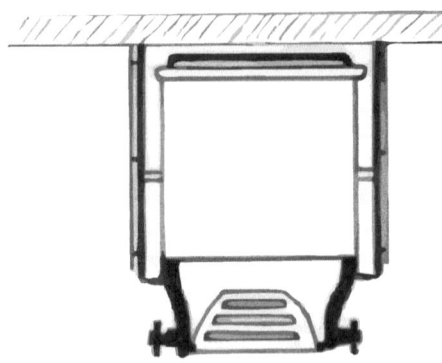

These bottom two diagrams show the chair against a wall. The bottom is the best as it is a big transfer, but you do get used to it. The trick is to not make a habit of falling out the chair, lol

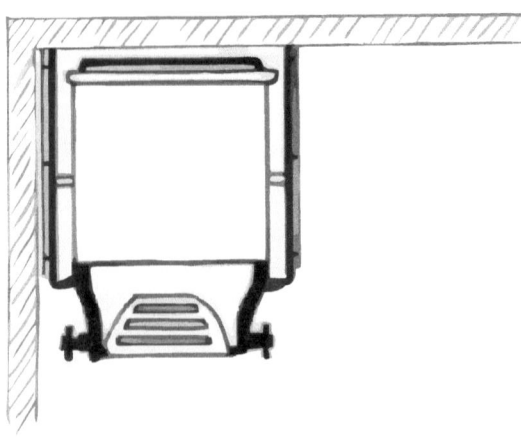

KITCHEN DIAGRAMS

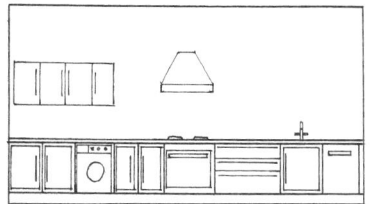
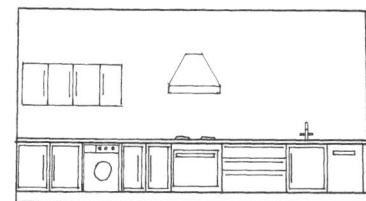

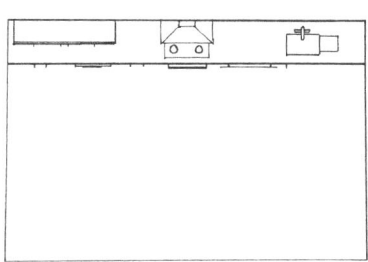
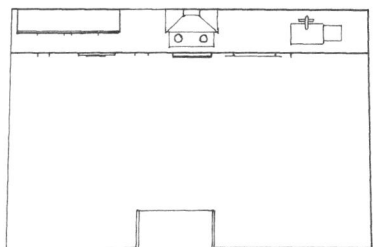

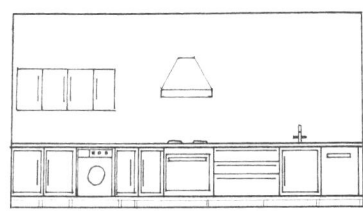
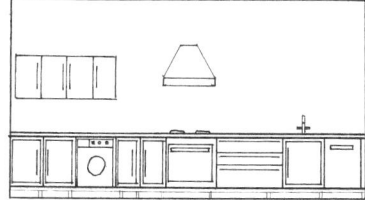

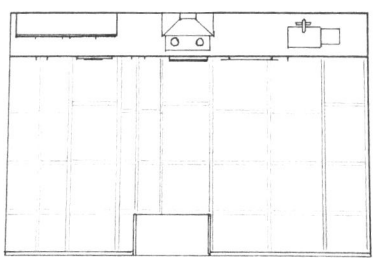
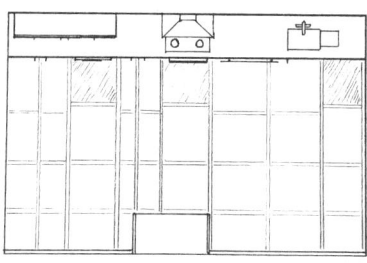

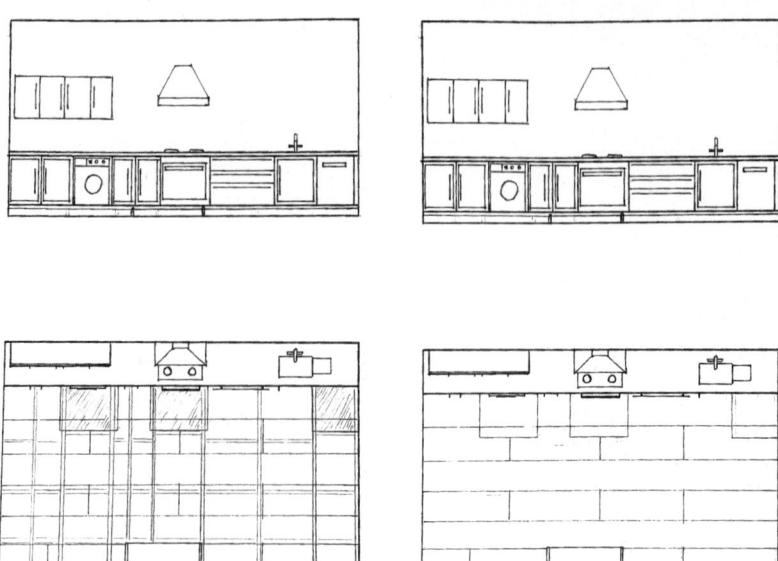

These are the diagrams I gave to the carpenter to illustrate the raised floor. All in it cost £400 and was good as I was still getting used to using a kitchen in a wheelchair. Also, the place I was living in was rented, so it was important to not make any permanent changes or risk damaging the floor etc.

HANDY GLOVES

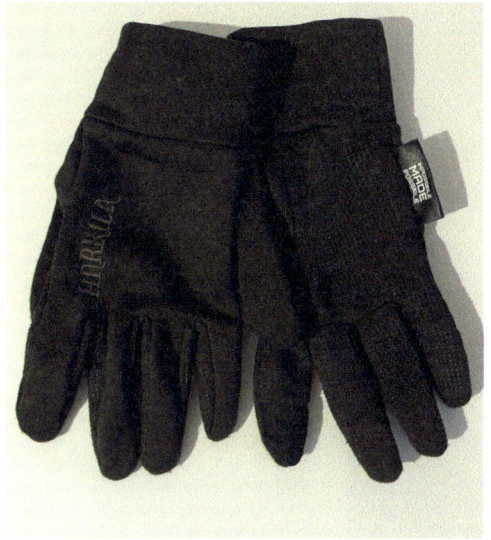 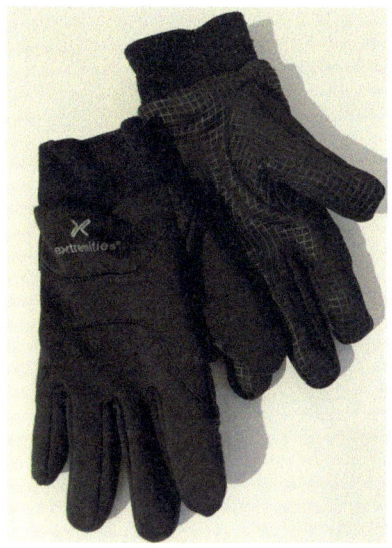

These are the thinner gloves which are more expensive but I use these mainly for shooting. The rubber grip on the inside is good when it is wet.

My every day gloves which cost about £11, but they last a good while and do keep my hands warm and again, they're good in the wet due to the rubber inside grips, so yes, handy!

29. SUMMARY

In all of this I have aimed to give you my personal view and approach as to how to live and cope with a disability with as much independence as possible. Hopefully in reading this it will help you to avoid some of the few (well, many) mistakes I've made.

This isn't a guidebook by any stretch of the imagination or a 'how to' book. It is just my views and thoughts based on the last ten years.

The journey you are now on is your own and I hope that this cuts the edges off some of the sharp learning curves I have had to face and that it helps you. I do understand everyone is different and I have tried to focus on having a disability rather than just a spinal cord injury which I have had so clearly I always fall back to that. But that is what landed me on wheels.

But the message I would say is that regardless of your disability or reason for being in a chair for a long while or shortish stretch is a simple one, you decide what you do at the end of the day. You can take all the advice in the world and look at various perspectives, but the main thing is you find your own level of happiness and peace.

At the end of the day we all have our problems, chair or not. Being able to talk about them openly and honestly is something that has taken me over ten year. I never pictured myself writing a book about it but I just felt it was time and I may have something to offer. If it helps just one person, then that's a job done.

And now it's time for the next chapter for me.. and you!

Whoever you are – the person in a chair, the friend, the partner, the family member, regardless I hope it helps and wish you well on your own path. God bless and good luck!

30. BACK OF THE BOOK: WHAT CAN YOU DO?

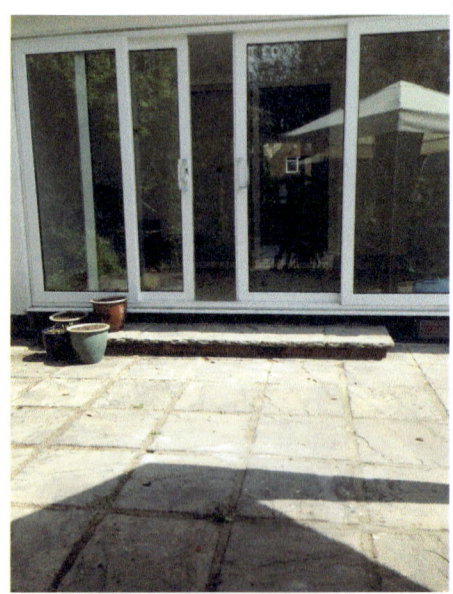
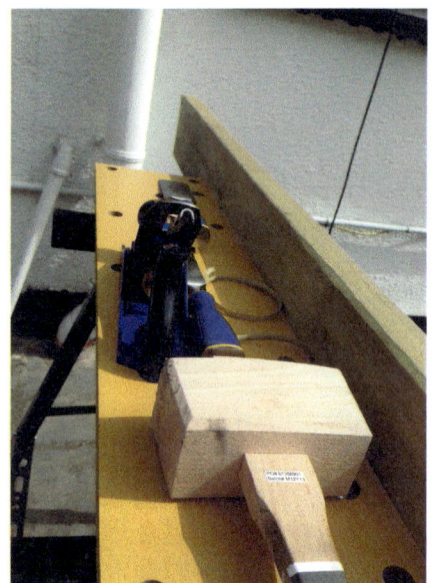
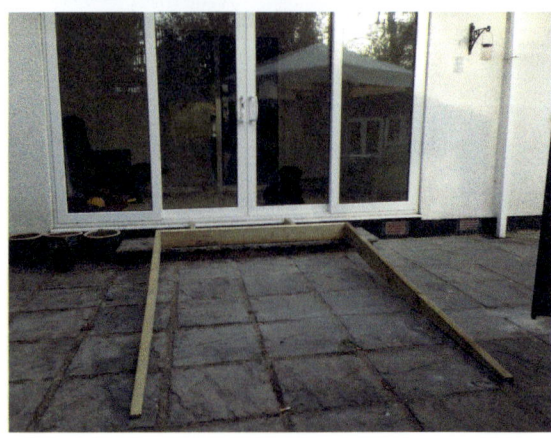
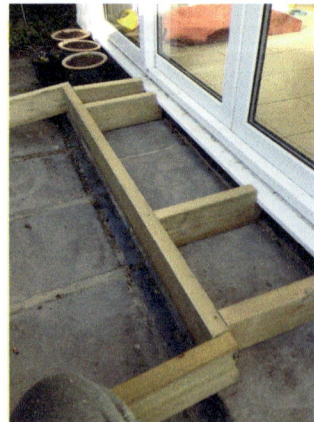

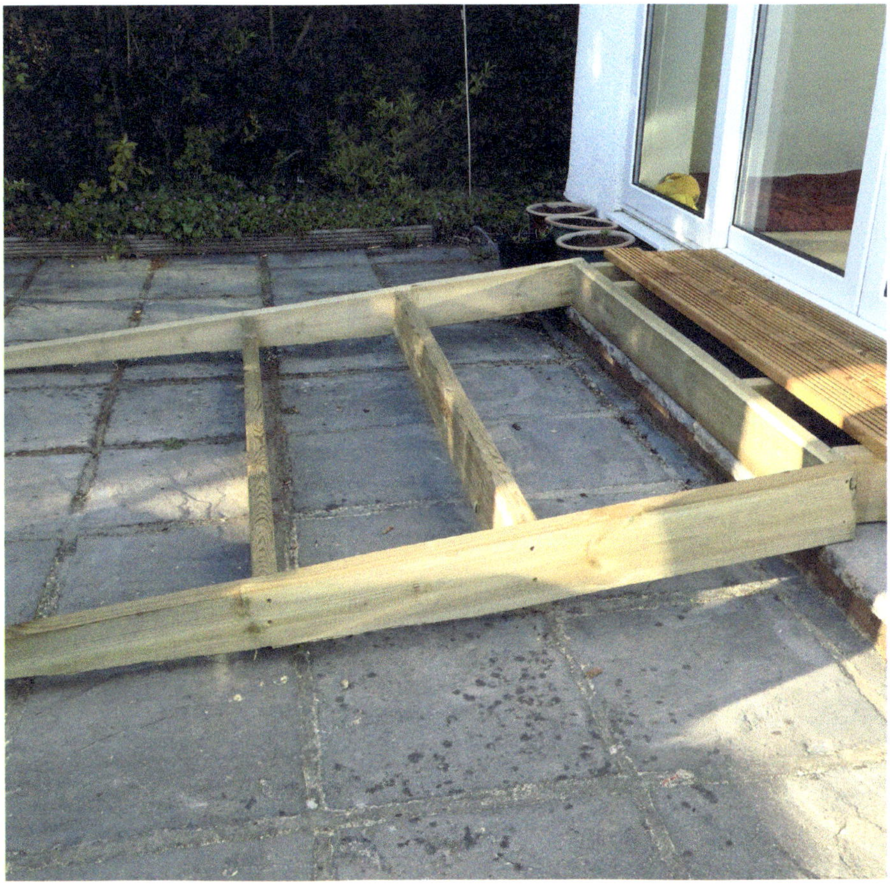

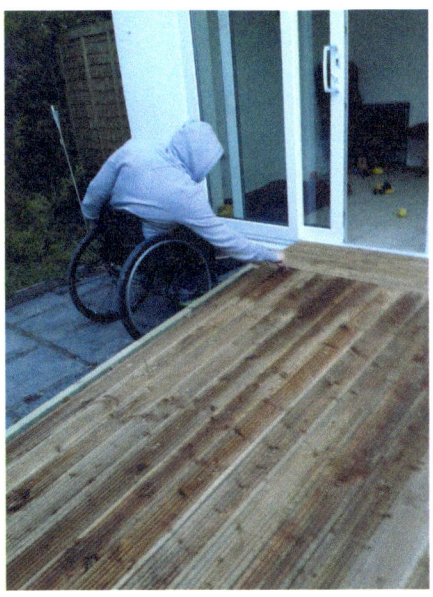
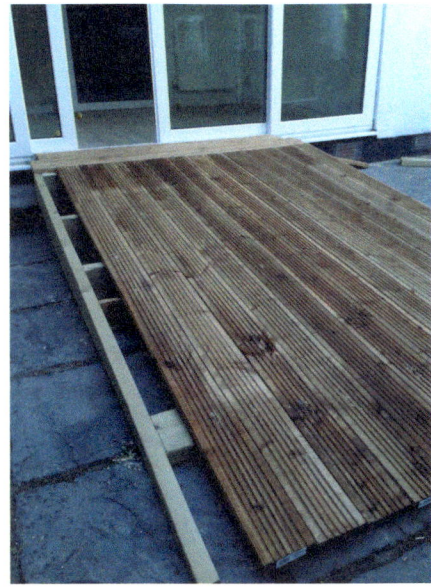

30. BACK OF THE BOOK: WHAT CAN YOU DO?

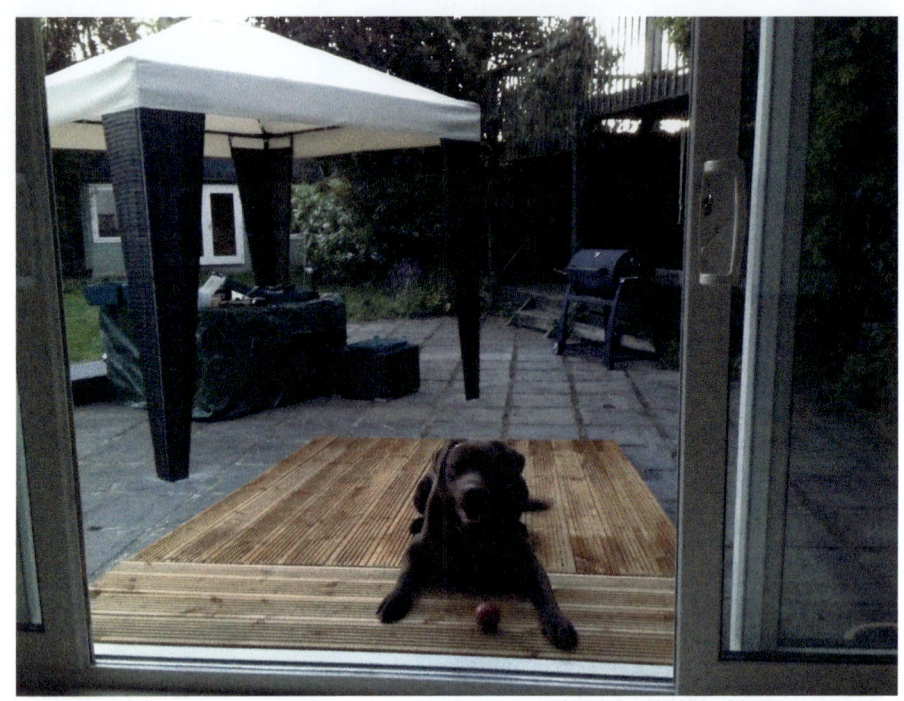
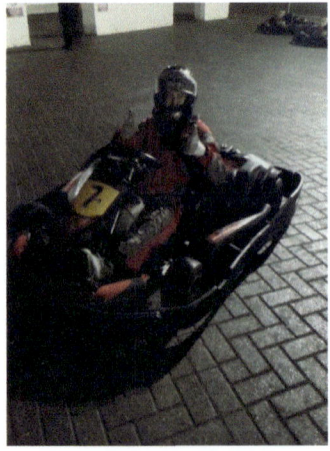
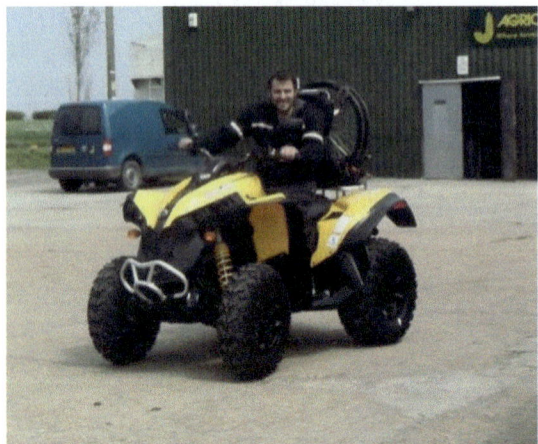

Just think what would you like to do then find a way there is always a way, to do what you enjoy and new things to try.

Best wishes

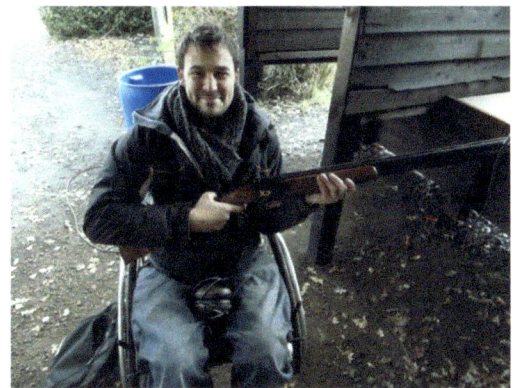
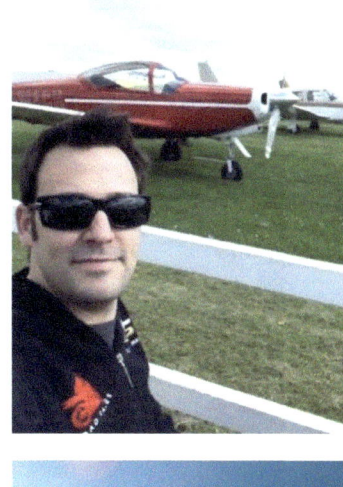
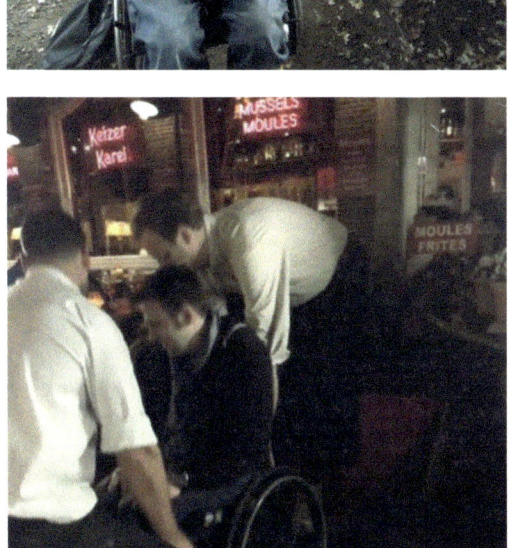
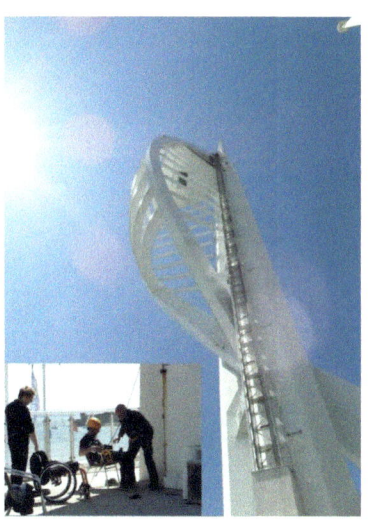
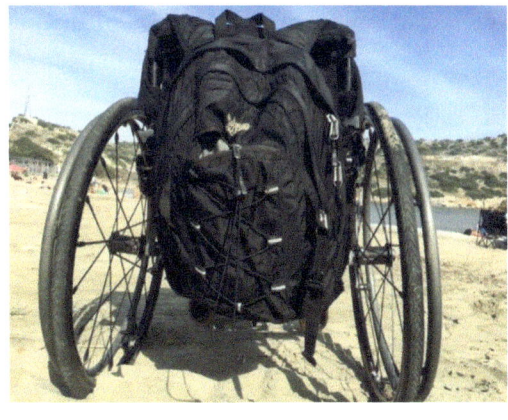
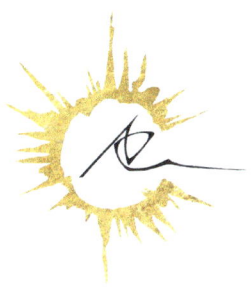

BV - #0083 - 240123 - C66 - 244/170/9 - PB - 9781913012908 - Matt Lamination